Lung Cancer

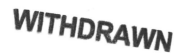

Lung Cancer

A Multidisciplinary Approach

Edited by
Alison Leary

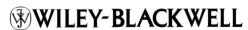

WILEY-BLACKWELL

A John Wiley & Sons, Ltd., Publication

This edition first published 2012 by Blackwell Publishing Ltd.
© 2012 by Blackwell Publishing Ltd.

Wiley-Blackwell is an imprint of John Wiley & Sons, formed by the merger of Wiley's global Scientific, Technical and Medical business with Blackwell Publishing.

Registered Office
John Wiley & Sons, Ltd, The Atrium, Southern Gate, Chichester, West Sussex, PO19 8SQ, UK

Editorial Offices
9600 Garsington Road, Oxford, OX4 2DQ, UK
The Atrium, Southern Gate, Chichester, West Sussex, PO19 8SQ, UK
2121 State Avenue, Ames, Iowa 50014-8300, USA

For details of our global editorial offices, for customer services and for information about how to apply for permission to reuse the copyright material in this book please see our website at www.wiley.com/wiley-blackwell.

Library of Congress Cataloging-in-Publication Data

Lung cancer : a multidisciplinary approach / edited by A. Leary.
    p. ; cm.
  Includes bibliographical references and index.
  ISBN 978-1-4051-8075-7 (pbk. : alk. paper)
I. Leary, A. (Alison), RN.
  [DNLM: 1. Lung Neoplasms. WF 658]
  616.99'424-dc23

                                2011035252

A catalogue record for this book is available from the British Library.

Wiley also publishes its books in a variety of electronic formats. Some content that appears in print may not be available in electronic books.

Set in 9/12.5pt Interstate Light by SPi Publisher Services, Pondicherry, India
Printed and bound in Singapore by Markono Print Media Pte Ltd

1 2012

Contents

Contributors   ix
Acknowledgements   xi

1 Introduction to Lung Cancer and Mesothelioma   **1**
Alison Leary

Introduction   1
Epidemiology and causes of lung cancer   2
Overview of the types of lung cancer   6
Delivering cancer services and the multidisciplinary team   8
Meeting information needs   11
Summary   13
References   13

**2 The Presentation and Diagnosis of Lung Cancer
and Mesothelioma**   **15**
Neal Navani and Stephen G. Spiro

Introduction   15
Clinical features of lung cancer   17
Paraneoplastic syndromes   22
Risk factors for lung cancer   26
Performance status   27
Investigation of lung cancer   28
Staging of lung cancer   38
An algorithm for the diagnosis and staging
    of non-small-cell lung cancer   41
Mesothelioma   42
Summary   46
References   46
Further reading   47

3 Chemotherapy and Biological Agents   **49**
Fharat A. Raja and Siow Ming Lee

Introduction   49
Chemotherapy   50
Chemotherapy for advanced NSCLC   53

Addition of targeted therapies to chemotherapy in NSCLC 55
Chemotherapy for small-cell lung cancer 57
Mesothelioma 59
Summary 61
References 61

4 Lung Radiotherapy **65**
Nita Patel and Dawn Carnell

Introduction 65
Principles of radiotherapy 65
The use of radiotherapy in non-small-cell lung cancer 73
The use of radiotherapy in small-cell lung cancer 76
Palliative radiotherapy 78
Management of patients during radiotherapy 80
New techniques under evaluation 83
Summary 84
References 84

5 Surgery for Lung Cancer **87**
Neil Cartwright and Aman S. Coonar

Introduction 87
The role of the surgeon 89
Reaching decisions about surgery 90
Surgery for cancers of the lung 100
The role of adjuvant treatment in NSCLC 108
Palliative surgical procedures 110
Carcinoid tumours and neuroendocrine cancer 111
Surgery for small-cell lung cancer 112
Bronchoalveolar cell cancer 112
Postoperative complications, rehabilitation follow-up 112
The multidisciplinary team in postsurgical care 115
Summary 116
References 116

6 The Nursing Care of Patients with Lung Cancer **121**
Sally Moore

Introduction 121
What are the important issues in relation to lung
 cancer nursing? 122
Context of lung cancer services 123
The challenges of lung cancer 124
The role of the specialist nurse 138
Summary 139
References 139

7   Supportive Care in Lung Cancer   **145**
Kay Eaton

Introduction   145
Supportive care   146
Communicating the 'diagnosis'   147
Attitudes towards cancer   148
Uncertainty   149
Psychological distress   150
A family-centred approach to care   152
Improving the patient experience: care across the pathway   153
Summary   156
References   156

8   End of Life Care   **159**
Michael Coughlan

Introduction   159
Palliative and end of life care   159
Dying in the twenty-first century   160
Diagnosing dying   162
Managing complex ethical dilemmas   163
Planning care for the patient dying from lung cancer   164
Summary   181
References   182

9   Quality of Life in Lung Cancer   **189**
Alison Leary

Introduction   189
Cancer: the journey, the individual and society   190
Doing the work of cancer and quality of life   192
Towards an understanding of the meaning
    of quality of life in lung cancer   192
Quality of life in advanced lung cancer: instruments
    used to measure health-related quality of life   197
Summary   199
References   199

Index   203

Contributors

Dawn Carnell, MB, BS, BSc, MRCP, FRCR
Consultant Clinical Oncologist, University College London
Hospitals NHS Foundation Trust, London, UK

Neil Cartwright, MA, MRCSEd, PhD
Specialty Registrar Cardiothoracic Surgery, Papworth
Hospital NHS Foundation Trust, Cambridge, UK

Aman S. Coonar, MD, MRCP, FRCS
Consultant Thoracic Surgeon, Papworth Hospital NHS Foundation Trust,
Cambridge, UK

Michael Coughlan, MSc, PG Dip, DPSN, RGN, RMN, FHEA
Programme Leader, Royal Marsden School of Cancer Nursing
and Rehabilitation, London, UK

Kay Eaton, MSc, RGN
Consultant Nurse in Cancer and Supportive Care, University College London
Hospitals NHS Foundation Trust, London, UK

Alison Leary, BSc Hons, MA, MSc, PhD, RN
Visiting Lecturer, Kings College London, London, UK

Siow Ming Lee, PhD, FRCP
Professor of Medical Oncology and Consultant Medical Oncologist,
University College London Hospitals NHS Foundation Trust, London, UK

Sally Moore, BSc (Hons), MSc, RGN
Nursing Research Fellow, Royal Marsden NHS Foundation Trust,
Surrey, UK

Neal Navani, MA, MRCP, MSc, PhD
Consultant in Thoracic Medicine, University College London Hospitals
NHS Foundation Trust, London, UK

Nita Patel, MBBS, BSc, MRCP (UK), FRCR
Consultant Clinical Oncologist, Guy's and St Thomas' Foundation Trust,
London, UK

Fharat A. Raja, BM, BCh, MRCP
Specialist Registrar, University College London Hospitals NHS Foundation Trust, London, UK

Stephen G. Spiro, BSc, MD, FRCP
Professor of Respiratory Medicine, Honorary Consultant, Royal Brompton and Harefield NHS Foundation Trust, London, UK

Acknowledgements

The Editor wishes to thank all of the contributing authors.

The book would not have been possible without the help and advice of many other experts in the field:

- Julia Solano and Linda Harvey, the Radiotherapy Service, University College London NHS Foundation Trust for their assistance.
- The Lung MDT at The Royal Brompton Hospital for the use of their image and for support.
- Maria Guerin and Liz Darlinson of the National Forum for Lung Cancer Nurses.
- The assistance of the press and media offices of Varian Medical Systems, Inc.
- Macmillan Cancer Support and the Cancer Research UK statistical team for the use of images.
- Angie Kyriacou and Rose Grant for their help in preparation of the manuscript.
- Jim McCarthy, Commissioning Editor.
- Magenta Styles and Alexandra McGregor from Wiley-Blackwell Publishers.
- Susan Oliver and Professor Jeffrey Tobias for their advice and encouragement.
- Professor Leonard Wutang as a sounding board for ideas.
- My friends and family for their tolerance, and especially Geoff Punshon for his ongoing support.

Alison Leary

Chapter 1

Introduction to Lung Cancer and Mesothelioma

Alison Leary

Key points

- Lung cancer is the most common cause of cancer worldwide and the most common cause of cancer death in the UK.
- The causes of lung cancer are multifactorial but there is a strong and established link with tobacco. Increasingly women who are never smokers are being diagnosed with lung cancer.
- Despite high levels of service improvement in cancer, there remains variability in the level of care provided to people with lung cancer.

Introducton

Malignant disease of the lung is a rare condition. The Middlesex Hospital Reports show only 890 cases of cancer of the Lung, 317 found at post mortem examination since records began.... As for prognosis a fatal termination is inevitable with average duration of the disease [life expectancy] to be 13.2 months.

Fowler and Rickman (1898), *Diseases of the Lung*

Lung cancer is currently the most common form of cancer worldwide...life expectancy is usually between three to seven months from diagnosis.

From Boyle *et al.* (2000), *Textbook of Lung Cancer*

From being a virtually unknown disease at the end of the nineteenth century, lung cancer has become the most common worldwide cancer. In just over 100 years lung cancer has become a modern epidemic. Thought to account for over 3 000 000 deaths each year worldwide and 33 400 deaths in the UK

Lung Cancer: A Multidisciplinary Approach, First Edition. Edited by Alison Leary.
© 2012 Blackwell Publishing Ltd. Published 2012 by Blackwell Publishing Ltd.

from the 39 000 diagnosed (Cancer Research UK (CRUK) 2010a) and with a 5-year survival rate of only 8–11% overall.

Five-year survival from lung cancer has barely improved in the last 30 years (Spiro and Silvestri 2005) but there has been a decline in deaths in the male population and an increase in female deaths. In contrast, 1-year survival has improved to some degree. In England and Wales 1-year survival in men with advanced non-small-cell lung cancer (NSCLC) rose from 15% in the 1970s to 25% in 2000/2001 (Coleman *et al.* 2004).

Average 5-year survival in the UK is 8.95%, which can be broken down by country:

- England (8.6%)
- Scotland (8.0%)
- Northern Ireland (10.2%)
- Wales (9.0%)

This is compared with 12.3% average in Europe (Berrino *et al.* 2007) and 15% in the USA (Reis *et al.* 2004). Surgical resection of lung cancer is the primary management, but the vast majority of patients with lung cancer present at a stage that is too advanced for surgery. Surgical resection rates are lower in the UK (11%) than Europe (17%) and North America (21%) (CRUK 2010a).

It is hoped that development of targeted therapies, earlier detection and increased opportunity for surgical intervention may improve the survival rate in lung cancer.

Epidemiology and causes of lung cancer

Until recently – as late as the 1990s – lung cancer was the most frequently occurring cancer in the UK. It has now been overtaken by breast cancer but is still the cause of 1 in 7 of all new cancer cases and 1 in 5 cancer deaths. In 2007, 39 473 people were diagnosed with lung cancer (CRUK 2010b). Most cases of lung cancer (approximately 86%) occur in people over the age of 60 years; the peaking age is 75–84 years (Fig. 1.1). Lung cancer accounts for 15% of all new male cancers and 12% of all new female cancers in the UK (CRUK 2010b). Lifetime risk of developing lung cancer is 1 in 14 for men and 1 in 21 for women in the UK.

Lung cancer incidence and social deprivation

Higher incidence of lung cancer has also been linked to areas associated with higher economic deprivation. Data from the 1990s shows that the incidence of lung cancer was thought to be three times higher in women in deprived areas and 2.5 times higher in men compared with the least-deprived areas (Fig. 1.2).

Lung cancer remains a cancer prevalent in areas of socioeconomic deprivation. Data from the National Cancer Intelligence Network (NCIN) in 2008 on

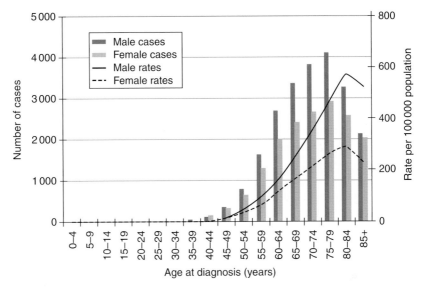

Fig. 1.1 Lung cancer: numbers of new cases and age-specific incidence rates by sex, UK 2007.
(*Source*: CRUK 2010b, reproduced with kind permission.)

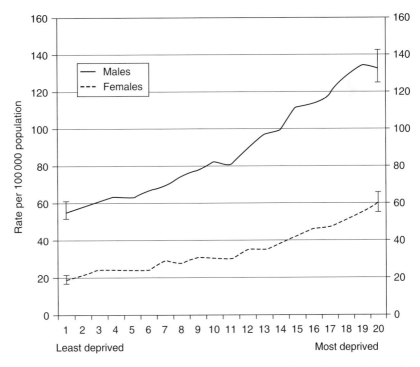

Fig. 1.2 Age-standardised incidence rates by deprivation category, England and Wales 1993.
(*Source*: CRUK 2010b, reproduced with kind permission.)

the years 2000-2004 demonstrated that if the incidence of lung cancer were the same in the most deprived groups as in the least deprived this would account for 11250 fewer cases of lung per year (NCIN 2008). Rates of lung cancer in Scotland are among the highest in the world, reflecting the history of high smoking prevalence. Many authors now comment that lung cancer is endemic in society (Boyle *et al.* 2000). The increase in incidence of lung cancer in the last hundred years has certainly been recognised. One of the causes of this rise is the now axiomatic link with smoking, particularly of tobacco.

Lung cancer incidence and smoking

From the mid-1950s there was an increase in the understanding of the aetiology of lung cancer and also the growing awareness that lung cancer was becoming more prevalent, reaffirming a causal link to smoking tobacco. This was in part due to the benchmark studies of Doll and Hill (1950, 1952, 1954). The body of evidence was so strong that in the USA the surgeon general was moved to produce an official statement on smoking and health that caused a worldwide reaction. After the publication of these documents, a more descriptive epidemiology of lung cancer occurred with the publishing of large cohort studies, for example the work of the National Cancer Institute in the USA.

From the 1960s onwards more epidemiological research into the rise of smoking-related diseases, of which non-small-cell lung cancer is just one, also charted the way in which smoking habits have changed. For example, in the 1970s consumers were made aware of tar levels and encouraged to smoke low-tar products. Some authors contend that this merely seems to have changed the histological subtype of lung cancer without reducing its incidence. Although tobacco smoking is thought to account for the majority of lung cancer deaths (CRUK 2010b) some authors, particularly from studies in the United States, cite as many as 10-20% of all newly diagnosed lung cancers being in those who have never smoked (never-smokers).

The link between lung cancer and smoking established in the 1950s and subsequent health promotion campaigns have influenced the public perception of lung cancer as a disease of smokers. In a recent survey by the UK Lung Cancer Coalition it was found that 40% of the population considered lung cancer to be a self-inflicted cancer, despite the fact that 1 in 8 lung cancer patients are never-smokers. The belief that lung cancer was a self inflicted cancer was higher (50%) in higher socioeconomic groups and lower (35%) in lower socioeconomic groups (UK Lung Cancer Coalition (UKLCC) 2005), and so whereas other patients with cancer are seen as victims by society, patients with lung cancer are seen as at least partly culpable for their disease. This then affects their perception of their own disease and some authors contend that lack of investment in research and other areas of lung cancer care stem from the less vocal nature of the lung cancer population and that as a group lung cancer patients tend to come from lower socioeconomic backgrounds with more limited access to education. Previous educational background influences how the cancer is perceived by the patient and family and also influences the subsequent information needs of the patient (Chapple *et al.* 2004; Jacobs-Lawson *et al.* 2009) Because of the established epidemiological link with tobacco use, lung cancer patients often experience feelings of stigmatisation and guilt (Chapple *et al.* 2004), which gives an added dimension to their suffering.

Lung cancer incidence and ethnicity

Data recently published by the National Cancer Intelligence Network on cancer incidence by survival in major ethnic group illustrates the difficulty of looking at ethnicity incidence. Data in this area is limited as it is only in recent years that routine data on ethnicity has been collected. However, from these data we can see that the rate of lung cancer in all non-white ethnic groups is significantly lower than in the white ethnic group, with people of all ages ranging from 23.1 to 37.2 per 100 000 in the Asian ethnic group, from 30.1 to 48.9 per 100 000 in the black ethnic group, from 22.4 to 48.6 per 100 000 in the Chinese ethnic group, and from 21.9 to 43.1 per 100 000 in the mixed ethnic group. In the white ethnic group the rate was 61.1 to 62.6 per 100 000 (NCIN 2009).

A standardised relative survival for the Asian ethnic group was significantly higher than the white ethnic group, for both 1 and 3 years; there is no significant difference in a standardised relative survival between black and white ethnic groups. For males aged 15–64 years at diagnosis, relative survival for the Asian ethnic group was significantly higher than for the white ethnic group at both 1 and 3 years. Given that the majority of lung cancers occur after the age of 60, these data have to be viewed in that context. For males aged 65–99 years, relative survival was significantly higher than in the white ethnic group for both Asian and black ethnic groups at both 1 and 3 years.

The causes of lung cancer

Although the link between smoking and lung cancer was established in the 1950s, the smoking or direct consumption of tobacco-related products is thought not to be the sole cause of lung cancer. It is estimated that exposure to passive smoking in the home causes around 11 000 deaths every year in the UK, from not only lung cancer but also stroke and ischaemic heart disease (CRUK 2010b).

Other causes of lung cancer are thought to include radon gas, which is a naturally occurring gas that increases the chance of developing lung cancer, particularly among smokers. Radon is present throughout the UK, but in some areas geological conditions can lead to higher than average levels. Some of the highest levels are found in the south west of England. Radon is thought to account for 50% of the exposure to radiation for the average UK adult (Health Protection Agency 2010) and thus is thought to contribute overall to the incidence of lung cancer.

Other risk factors for lung cancer include industrial carcinogens; for example, arsenic, asbestos, polycyclic hydrocarbons or nonferrous metals. More recently, air pollution is now also thought to make a small contribution to the lung cancer risk burden. There is some evidence to suggest that an increase in risk of lung cancer caused by exposure to nitrogen oxides, particularly those in traffic fumes (Vineis *et al.* 2006). Despite these other risk factors, smoking remains the largest one. Current smokers are 15 times more likely to die from lung cancer than lifelong non-smokers. The risk of developing lung cancer is affected by the level of consumption and the length of time for which a person has smoked.

Overview of the types of lung cancer

Lung cancer is divided broadly into two types; non-small-cell lung cancer (NSCLC) and small-cell lung cancer (SCLC). Non-small-cell lung cancers were historically grouped together as treatment offered was often the same for each type of NSCLC but different from that for SCLC. Increasingly, however, NSCLC is thought of as much more variable. It has three main variants and this is reflected in the different treatment regimes, survival rates and range of symptoms on presentation.

In addition, another disease affecting the lung, but not a primary tumour of the bronchus or lung tissue, is malignant pleural mesothelioma (MPM). Mesothelioma can affect the pleura or peritoneum and is often managed by the same multidisciplinary team as those with lung cancer.

Non-small-cell lung cancers (NSCLC)

Non-small-cell lung cancers are divided broadly into three types by histology. This was because historically all non-small-cell lung cancer patients were offered a limited set of treatment options. Now, with new agents and the increasingly precise nature of staging of this cancer in recent years, this has changed and is explored in more detail in Chapters 2 and 3.

Most of the patients who present with NSCLC do so as a result of progression of the tumour either locally in the chest or by metastatic spread. Such progression can precipitate the symptoms of dyspnoea, cough, chronic respiratory illness, haemoptysis and pain. Direct tumour invasion to the left laryngeal nerve may cause hoarseness of voice as a presenting symptom. Other presenting symptoms may be due to the spread of distant metastases; for example, pain at the site of bone metastasis.

The following are the main histological groupings of non-small-cell lung cancer.

- **Squamous** cell carcinoma is the most common type, accounting for 20–25% of lung cancers. Squamous cell carcinoma is usually a tumour arising from bronchial squamous epithelium and has several variants. It is the most common lung cancer in smokers.
- **Adenocarcinoma** of the lung arises from the secretory (glandular) cells located in the epithelium lining the bronchi. It is increasing in incidence and

it is likely to surpass squamous cell carcinoma in the near future as the most common type of NSCLC. Although adenocarcinoma occurs often in smokers, it is becoming the more prevalent variant of NSCLC in non-smokers and is also becoming the most common type of lung cancer in women. It can arise centrally or in the lung periphery.

- **Large-cell carcinoma** is composed of large-sized cells that are anaplastic and often arise in the bronchi.

In addition there are also bronchoalveolar carcinoma and others variants such as mixed and undifferentiated pulmonary carcinomas. It is more common these days to pursue the subtype of NSCLC histology as this can now inform treatment decisions. It is not uncommon to find mixed histological subtypes in lung cancer.

Around 80% of lung cancers in the UK are non-small-cell lung cancers (CRUK 2010b).

Small-cell lung cancer (SCLC)

Small-cell lung cancer (also known as oat cell) is a primary lung cancer that usually arises centrally in the chest (large airways or lymph nodes). It makes up the reminder of primary lung cancers in the UK.

SCLC is associated with paraneoplastic syndromes at presentation such as inappropriate secretion of antidiuretic hormone (ISADH) as small-cell tumours contain dense neurosecretory granules that can then give this tumour endocrine/paraneoplastic syndrome components. SCLC is generally more sensitive to chemotherapy and radiation, but it often presents with metastasis in areas such as the brain or liver and usually carries a worse prognosis. Small-cell lung cancers have traditionally been staged into limited and extensive stage disease. There is recent research, however, to revise the staging system for SCLC (Shepherd 2007). This type of lung cancer is strongly associated with smoking.

Carcinoid tumours

Carcinoid tumours are occasionally found in the lung and have been defined by the World Health Organisation (Solcia et al. 2000). They are divided into typical and atypical and can grow either in the airways or the lung periphery. Like SCLC, carcinoid tumours are neuroendocrine tumours and can present with local signs and symptoms such as haemoptysis or systemic symptoms such as carcinoid syndromes (flushing, wheezing, shortness of breath, tachycardia). The most common site of carcinoid tumours is the gastrointestinal tract, but occasionally they occur in the lung. Resection is the primary means of treatment.

Malignant pleural mesothelioma

Mesothelioma is a cancer of the mesothelium and peritoneum; the most common form of this is pleural mesothelioma, also known as malignant pleural mesothelioma or MPM. Pleural mesothelioma causes the pleura to thicken.

Lung expansion can become compromised and pleural effusion, pain, weight loss or breathlessness can be some of the presenting symptoms.

Approximately 2000 people are diagnosed with mesothelioma in the UK each year (Macmillan Cancer Support 2010). In pleural mesothelioma the pleura thicken and it is thought that exposure to asbestos is responsible for 90% of all mesothelioma cases (Mesothelioma UK 2010).

Delivering cancer services and the multidisciplinary team

The years since the late 1990s have seen significant changes in the way cancer services in the UK are delivered. A programme of investment and reform with the aim of equitable and timely care delivery has taken place, with significant investment in cancer care. A fundamental part of this reform was the launch in 2000 by the Department of Health (DH) of the NHS Cancer Plan (DH 2000). The NHS Cancer Plan essentially had four aims: to save more lives; to ensure that people with cancer got the right professional support and care as well as the best treatments; to tackle the inequalities in health that mean unskilled workers are twice as likely to die from cancer as professionals; and 'to build for the future for investment in the cancer workforce through strong research and through the preparation for the genetics revolution so that the NHS never falls behind on cancer care again' (DH 2000).

In the 10 years in which the NHS Cancer Plan was launched in England there was significant improvement in the way services were delivered. One of the most significant changes was the assurance that implementation of the plan would reduce waiting times for diagnosis and treatment of any cancer. The NHS Cancer Plan recognised the inequalities in cancer care in England and became a foundation to its improvement. In 2007 the Department of Health published the Cancer Reform Strategy (DH 2007). This work reviewed the progress of the Cancer Plan with the aim of increasing cancer prevention, further speeding up the diagnosis and treatment of cancer, continuing to reduce inequalities, improving the experience of people living with and beyond cancer, ensuring that care is delivered in the most appropriate setting, and ensuring that patients can access effective new treatments quickly (DH 2007).

Many of the improvements made as a result of cancer reform in England are now included in the NHS Constitution. This includes the pledge of a maximum two-week wait to see a specialist referred for suspected cancer by their GP and that all patients referred with a suspected cancer by their GP will wait no more than 62 days from referral to treatment.

Despite many improvements in cancer care as a result of these initiatives, the recent National Lung Cancer Audit (NHS IC 2009) demonstrated that, although there have been improvements in lung cancer care, there is still variation in services offered. For example, nationally 54% of patients with lung cancer were offered an anti-cancer treatment (chemotherapy, radiotherapy, surgery) in 2008 but this varied between hospital trusts and was as low as

10% in some trusts (range 10–80%). Thus, some inequalities remain in the provision of good lung cancer care.

The complexity of cancer care

The delivery of cancer care in the UK is necessarily complex despite the reforms. To achieve a high level of cancer care requires the involvement of many different professionals and sometimes the resources of one or more treatment centres. To improve efficiency in cancer services, cancer pathways were streamlined, particularly at the start of the this century. Although this has made pathways more efficient and easier for patients to understand, there is still a considerable amount of work involved on the part of the patient and the service provider to navigate these pathways. There are many steps inherent in reaching a diagnosis and then a treatment plan, and patients have to deal with this as work when they also understand that they are being investigated for a cancer diagnosis. This adds to the stress and suffering experienced by people undergoing this process and for this reason much has been done to streamline the process and remove the burden of work from the patient and family. In addition, access to a specialist cancer nurse who can clarify this pathway, provide support and meet information needs is essential.

Recent cancer improvement initiatives have seen the focus of cancer move towards patient-centred care. The NICE 2005 guidance (NICE 2005 updated 2011) on lung cancer states that good communication between healthcare professionals and patients is essential and should be supported by the provision of evidence-based information offered in a form that is tailored to meet the needs of the individual patient. Current cancer patients are cared for by a multidisciplinary team (MDT) of professionals, each with a distinctive professional background and role, who are then able to offer optimum treatments, support and care to those patients. Lung cancer is no exception to this, and lung cancer patients should now be cared for by a MDT. The core members of the MDT include oncologists, chest physicians, specialist nurses, radiologists, pathologists and surgeons. To help patients navigate the complexity particularly around the diagnosis phase of lung cancer, patients are offered a 'key worker'; this usually is a clinical nurse specialist in lung cancer who acts as a key accessible professional with the knowledge to meet the patient's information needs while negotiating a complex pathway. These teams meet on a weekly basis to discuss new patients and any ongoing care issues (Fig. 1.3).

Members of the core lung cancer MDT are:

- Medical oncologists (who normally specialise in chemotherapy and other agents)
- Clinical oncologists (who normally specialise in radiation treatments)
- Chest physician
- Clinical nurse specialist in lung cancer

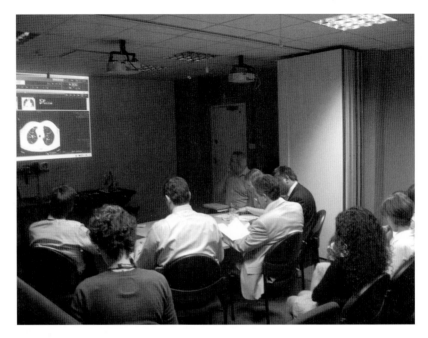

Fig. 1.3 A multidisciplinary team meeting.

- Surgeons (thoracic or cardiothoracic)
- A palliative care clinician
- Radiologists including interventional radiologists
- Pathologists (cytologist and histopathologist)
- MDT coordinator who tracks patients in the pathway and organises the investigations. Many MDT coordinators will work with the clinical nurse specialist to facilitate proactive case management.
- Research nurse/coordinator

The extended members of the team can also include:

- Other specialist nurses (e.g. chemotherapy specialists)
- Physiotherapists
- Occupational therapists
- Dieticians
- Speech and language therapists
- Therapy radiographers
- Spiritual/chaplaincy representatives
- Psychologists
- Counsellors
- Complementary therapists
- Benefits advisors
- Social workers

The role of the MDT coordinator

The MDT coordinator tracks patients in the pathway and organises the investigations. Many MDT coordinators will work with the clinical nurse specialist to facilitate proactive case management.

Many MDT coordinators are also responsible for collecting much of the data required to run an efficient cancer service.

The role of the clinical nurse specialist

A clinical nurse specialist is a nurse who has a substantial role in the care of the lung cancer or mesothelioma patient. The clinical nurse specialist is often the member of the team responsible for case management.

Clinical nurse specialists:

- Use and apply complex technical knowledge of lung cancer and treatment to meet the complex information and support needs of patients and their families.
- Act as the accessible professional for the multidisciplinary team, allowing patients and carers faster access to an expert at any point in the cancer journey.
- Undertake proactive case management and use clinical acumen and expertise to reduce the risk to patients from disease or treatments, for example by recognizing signs of illness or recurrence.
- Use empathy, knowledge and experience to assess and alleviate the psychosocial suffering of cancer by providing psychological interventions/counselling. These interventions may include referring to other agencies or disciplines as appropriate. This will for most lung cancer patients include a transition into palliative care, perhaps with input from a specialist palliative care team.
- Use technical knowledge and insight from patient experience to lead service redesign in order to implement improvements and make services responsive to patient need.

Nursing care of patients with lung cancer is described in Chapter 6.

Work done by the UK Lung Cancer Coalition (UKLCC 2008) showed that the MDT was having a positive impact on lung cancer care, with greater access for patients to a variety of appropriate treatments.

Meeting information needs

One of the ways cancer patients alleviate some of the uncertainty and suffering of the cancer diagnosis period is to seek information. This information must be of good quality and accessible to the patient. The range of patient information available is varied, from disease-specific information to

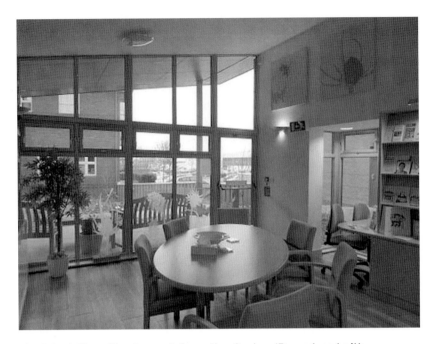

Fig. 1.4 A Macmillan Cancer Information Centre. (Reproduced with permission of Macmillan Cancer support.)

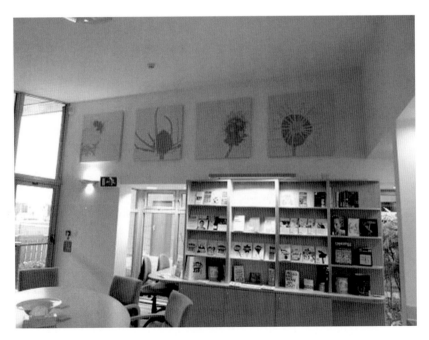

Fig. 1.5 Examples of written information on offer in a cancer information centre. (Reproduced with permission of Macmillan Cancer support.)

information on diagnostic procedures, treatment regimes such as chemotherapy, financial advice and information on subjects such as dealing with fatigue or coping emotionally with the diagnosis and treatment of cancer. Because the range of information is so broad, many cancer networks now advocate the use of information pathways whereby information can be given out at appropriate times in the pathway, always supported by the clinicians helping the patient to interpret the information. In addition to this, some charities such as Macmillan have now set up cancer information centres (Fig. 1.4) in hospitals and other areas where cancer patients may be treated to help patients through the various stages of the cancer journey. These centres offer a range of printed information (Fig. 1.5) and can also signpost to other services such as benefits advice or complementary therapies.

Summary

Lung cancer is endemic in society. Five-year survival is still poor but 1-year survival is improving. Greater understanding of lung cancer as a disease has lead to newer more targeted therapies. The largest risk factor of lung cancer is smoking and it is likely that the most effective way to tackle lung cancer is smoking cessation. Lung cancer disproportionately affects those from deprived backgrounds and this inequality needs to be addressed.

Cancer services and the way that cancer care is delivered have improved over the first ten years of this century as part of the NHS modernisation agenda, but the delivery of lung cancer services is still variable in some areas. All cancer care should be managed by an MDT to give patients the optimum treatment options and supportive care.

References

Berrino, F., De Angelis, R., Sant, M., *et al.* (2007) Survival for eight major cancers and all cancers combined for European adults diagnosed in 1995–99: results of the EUROCARE-4 study. *The Lancet Oncology*, **8** (9), 752–753.

Boyle, P., Gandini, S., and Grey, N. (2000) Epidemiology of lung cancer: a century of great success and ignominious failure. In: *Textbook of Lung Cancer* (ed. H. Hansen). Martin Dunitz, London.

Chapple, A., Ziebland, S., and McPherson, A. (2004) Stigma, shame and blame experienced by patients with lung cancer: qualitative study. *British Medical Journal*, **328** (7454), 1470. doi:10.1136/bmj.38111.639734.7c. 2004.

Coleman, M.P., Rachet, B., and Woods, L. (2004) Trends and socioeconomic inequalities in cancer survival in England and Wales to 2001. *British Journal of Cancer*, **90** (7), 1367–1373.

CRUK (2010a) Regional variation in survival rates. Cancer Research UK, London. Available at http://info.cancerresearchuk.org/cancerstats/types/lung/survival/index.htm. Accessed May 2010.

CRUK (2010b) Incidence statistics (lung cancer). Cancer Research UK, London. Available at http://info.cancerresearchuk.org/cancerstats/types/lung/incidence/index.htm. Accessed May 2010.

DH (Department of Health) (2000) *The NHS Cancer Plan: A plan for investment, a plan for reform*. HMSO, London.

DH (Department of Health) (2007) *Cancer Reform Strategy*. HMSO, London.

Doll, R. and Hill, A.B. (1950) Smoking and carcinoma of the lung. *British Medical Journal*, Sept. 30, **2** (4682), 739–748.

Doll, R. and Hill, A.B. (1952) A study of the aetiology of carcinoma of the lung. *British Medical Journal*, Dec. 13, **2** (4797), 1271–1286.

Doll, R. and Hill, A.B. (1954) The mortality of doctors in relation to their smoking habits. *British Medical Journal*, Jun 26, **1** (4877), 1451–1455.

Fowler, J.K. and Rickman, J.G. (1898) *Diseases of the Lungs*. Longman Greene, London.

Health Protection Agency (2010) Radon at a glance. HPA, London. Available at http://www.hpa.org.uk/Topics/Radiation/UnderstandingRadiation/UnderstandingRadiationTopics/Radon/. Accessed May 2010.

Jacobs-Lawson, J.M., Scumacher, M.M., Hughes, T., and Arnold. S. (2009) The relationship between lung cancer patients' educational level and evaluation of their treatment information needs. *Journal of Cancer Education*, **24** (4), 346–350.

Macmillan Cancer Support (2010) *Understanding Lung Cancer*. Macmillan Cancer Support, London.

Mesothelioma UK (2010) Mesothelioma information. Avaialble at http://www.mesothelioma.uk.com/index.php?pageno=18. Accessed May 2010.

National Institute for Clinical Excellence (NICE) and National Collaborating Centre for Acute Care (2005) *The Diagnosis and Treatment of Lung Cancer*. NICE London.

NCIN (2008) *Cancer Incidence by Deprivation England, 1995-2004*. National Cancer Intelligence Network. Available at http://library.ncin.org.uk/docs/081202-NCIN-incidence_by_Deprivation_95_04.pdf. Accessed May 2010.

NCIN (2009) *Cancer Incidence and Survival by Major Ethnic Group, England, 2002 - 2006*. National Cancer Intelligence Network. http://library.ncin.org.uk/docs/090625-NCIN-Incidence_and_Survival_by_Ethnic_Group-Report.pdf. Accessed May 2010.

NHS IC (2009) *National Lung Cancer Audit*. The NHS Information Centre, London.

Shepherd, F., Crowley, J., Van Houtte, P., *et al.* (2007) The International Association for the Study of Lung Cancer Lung Cancer Staging Project: Proposals Regarding the Clinical Staging of Small-Cell Lung Cancer in the Forthcoming (Seventh) Edition of the Tumor, Node, Metastasis Classification for Lung Cancer. *Journal of Thoracic Oncology*, **2** (12), 1067–1077.

Solcia, E., Kloppel, G., Sobin, L.H., *et al.* (2000) Histologic typing of endocrine tumours. *WHO International Histological Classification of Tumours*. Springer Verlag, Heidelberg.

Spiro, S.G. and Silvestri, G.A. (2005) One hundred years of lung cancer. *American Review of Respiratory Critical Care Medicine*, **172** (5), 523–529.

UKLCC (2005) *Lung Cancer Awareness Survey*. UK Lung Cancer Coalition. Available at http://www.uklcc.org.uk/word/uklccresearchfactsheet.doc. Accessed May 2010.

UKKLCC (2008) *Is Your MDT Fit for Purpose?* Report from The International Lung Cancer Conference. UK Lung Cancer Coalition. Available at http://www.uklcc.org.uk/pdf/UKLCC%20MDT%20Report%20FINAL%20Oct%2008.pdf. Accessed May 2010.

Vineis, P., Hoek, G., Krzyzanowski, M., *et al.* (2006) Air pollution risk of lung cancer in a prospective study in Europe. *International Journal of Cancer*, **119**, 169–174.

Chapter 2

The Presentation and Diagnosis of Lung Cancer and Mesothelioma

Neal Navani and Stephen G. Spiro

Key points

- Symptoms occur late in the natural history of lung cancer and therefore the majority of lung cancers present with advanced disease.
- The symptoms and signs of lung cancer may arise from the primary lesion, metastatic spread, constitutional effects or paraneoplastic syndromes.
- The disease stage and the patient's performance status guide treatment options.

Introduction

Although it remains more common in men than women, incidence rates of lung cancer for men in the UK have fallen by 20% between 1997 and 2006, reflecting the decrease in smoking rates in men since the 1970s. Female lung cancer rates, however, have increased by 10% in the same period. As well as a shift in gender of the epidemiology of lung cancer, there may also have been a change in the global distribution of disease. Effective anti-smoking campaigns have seen a decline in the number of lung cancers in industrialised countries. Currently, central and eastern Europe experience the highest incidence for men, with rates for women highest in North America. As smoking increases in developing countries, the burden of disease of this largely preventable cancer is likely to spread to these newer nations. Lung cancer is already responsible for 600 000 deaths per year in China and this figure is predicted to rise.

Lung Cancer: A Multidisciplinary Approach, First Edition. Edited by Alison Leary.
© 2012 Blackwell Publishing Ltd. Published 2012 by Blackwell Publishing Ltd.

Table 2.1 Natural history of untreated lung cancer.

Cell type	Volume doubling time (days)	Time from malignant change (years)		
		Earliest diagnosis	Usual diagnosis	Death
Diameter		1 cm	3 cm	10 cm
Small-cell	20–50	2.4	2.8	3.2
Squamous	80–100	7.1	8.4	9.6
Adenocarcinoma	150–175	13.2	15.4	17.6

Adapted from Geddes (1979).

Unfortunately, lung cancer is usually recognised late in its natural history, so that curative treatment is rarely possible. This reflects the fact that the presentation of lung cancer potentially exhibits two main problems. Firstly, the anatomy of the thorax allows a tumour to grow for a considerable period of time before symptoms arise; and secondly, the symptoms of lung cancer, when they do occur, are often non-specific (e.g. cough). Lung parenchyma (and visceral pleura) are equipped with afferent C fibres that relay stretch sensations only and so intra-parenchymal lesions often remain asymptomatic, since there are no pain fibres within the lungs. The doubling time of untreated lung cancer ranges from 29 days for the small-cell type to 161 days for adeno-carcinoma (Table 2.1). By the time a tumour (originating as a single cell) has doubled 20 times, it is 1 mm in diameter yet presents on average at 3–4 cm in diameter on chest radiography. Therefore, lung cancers are often asympto-matic for much of their natural history and by the time they are detected the patient has advanced disease that is beyond cure. These observations explain why the curative surgery rate for lung cancer in the UK is only between 10% and 20% and 5-year survival is as low as 7%.

The non-specific and vague presentation of lung cancer may also be responsible for the delay from the patient's first experiencing symptoms to their seeking medical attention. This varies from 3 weeks to 3 months. A Swedish study of 134 patients found that the mean delay from first symp-tom to presentation was 43 days. Efforts have been directed at encouraging patients to present sooner (e.g. Lung Cancer Awareness Month). However, in the context of lung cancer doubling times, it is unclear what impact this will have on outcome.

Given the insidious and late presentation of lung cancer, patients who have the disease detected incidentally have a better prognosis. Increasingly, imag-ing with chest radiography (chest X-ray: CXR) or computed tomography (CT) is carried out for other reasons, without a clinical suspicion of lung cancer. An asymptomatic lung cancer detected by chance is less likely to have spread and therefore may be more amenable to curative treatment. Indeed, the 5-year survival for patients who are asymptomatic at presentation is 18%. These arguments form the basis for lung cancer screening in selected populations, which will be discussed in more detail elsewhere.

Clinical features of lung cancer

The majority of patients with lung cancer have symptoms at presentation. However, the symptoms and signs are difficult to distinguish from those of other common pathological processes. Furthermore, the most common symptoms are often constitutional and reflect metastatic disease, rendering the patient inoperable at presentation. Establishing the history remains crucial in developing rapport with the patient, elucidating concerns, determining patient fitness (performance status) and arriving at the diagnosis and treatment plan.

Symptoms and signs of intrapulmonary disease

- Cough is the most common symptom of a primary tumour and may be found in up to 75% of patients presenting with lung cancer (Table 2.2). However, the vast majority of patients with cough do not have lung cancer. In a Dutch study of 11000 encounters over 10 years of patients with a cough, lung cancer was not even listed separately in the top 20 common diagnoses. Only 3% of the consultations were due to lung cancer. A *change* in cough or sputum production may be a more specific symptom and this should always be taken seriously and prompt investigation by at least CXR. Copious sputum production may be consistent with bronchoalveolar carcinoma, a rare lung cancer cell type (3% of all lung cancers).
- Haemoptysis is the only symptom that consistently prompts more urgent presentation and may occur in up to 35% of cases of lung cancer. Haemoptysis has a wide differential diagnosis, including infection, but nearly always warrants further investigation. It is recommended that patients over the age of 40 years and with a significant smoking history (>20 pack years) undergo more detailed investigations. Patients with haemoptysis due to lung cancer commonly have an abnormal CXR but even if a radiograph is within normal limits there is still a 5–10% chance of finding an endobronchial lesion at bronchoscopy.
- Chest pain in the form of a vague, heavy, central discomfort may persist for weeks before the patient seeks medical advice. More severe pain may be caused by direct extension of the primary tumour into the parietal pleura and chest wall.
- A recurrent focal pneumonia or one that fails to resolve with appropriate treatment should also prompt the search for an obstructing endobronchial lesion.

Table 2.2 Frequency of initial symptoms and signs of lung cancer.

Symptoms and signs	Range of frequency (%)
Cough	8–75
Weight loss	0–68
Dyspnoea	3–60
Chest pain	20–49
Haemoptysis	6–35
Bone pain	6–25
Clubbing	0–20
Fever	0–20
Hoarseness	2–18
Weakness	0–10
Superior vena cava obstruction	0–4
Dysphagia	0–2
Wheezing and stridor	0–2

Adapted from Spiro et al. (2007).

- Breathlessness is an important symptom of lung cancer in up to 60% of patients and may result from excess sputum production and cough or occlusion of a main airway causing monophonic wheeze. This may progress to complete occlusion of the main airway with distal collapse and the accompanying clinical signs of reduced expansion and dullness to percussion over the collapsed lobe. Breathlessness in a lung cancer patient may also be due to pleural or pericardial effusions, pulmonary embolic disease, lymphangitis carcinomatosa or compression of the pulmonary vessels by tumour.
- Tracheal obstruction is a life-threatening complication of lung cancer that is rare but important as it is nearly always mistaken for asthma or chronic obstructive pulmonary disease (COPD) initially. Its onset is gradual but progressive and patients may complain of breathlessness and have evidence of inspiratory stridor. The peak expiratory flow (PEF) is disproportionately reduced in patients with tracheal obstruction when compared with the forced expiratory volume in 1 second (FEV_1), such that the ratio of the FEV_1 (in mL) to the PEF (in L/min) is greater than 10. This simple bedside assessment may identify impending upper airway obstruction.

Symptoms and signs of extrapulmonary intrathoracic disease

Intrathoracic spread of lung cancer from the lung itself may occur by direct extension of the primary tumour or from lymphatic or vascular spread. Any of the structures within the thoracic cage may be involved, resulting in a wide variety of symptoms and signs.

- Superior vena caval obstruction (SVCO) is one of the more dramatic and is caused by lung cancer in up to 75% of cases, with small-cell lung cancer being the predominant tissue type. Right upper lobe tumours or adjacent metastatic right paratracheal nodes compress or invade the superior vena cava. The patient may complain of headaches, blurred vision, facial fullness on bending over, and breathlessness due to extrinsic tracheal compression. Examination may reveal facial plethora, oedema, persistently elevated jugular venous pressure and dilated superficial collateral veins over the upper chest, arms, rib cage and abdomen. The symptoms and signs may develop relatively swiftly over the course of a few weeks and should prompt immediate referral to secondary care. Unless collateral circulation opens up, sudden death can occur.

- Horner syndrome result from direct extension of an apical or Pancoast tumour into the superior sympathetic chain. This causes ipsilateral ptosis (due to interruption of the preganglionic sympathetic supply to the Muller muscle of the eyelid), meiosis, enophthalmos and anhidrosis. The brachial plexus and in particular nerve roots C8, T1 and T2 are situated in direct proximity to the posterior aspect of the lung apex and are vulnerable to direct invasion by Pancoast tumours. Initially, this may cause shoulder and neck pain. However as the tumour progresses, weakness, atrophy and par-aesthesias of the hand, forearm and arm may develop. Wasting of the small muscles of the hand may be particularly debilitating for the patient and is an important clinical sign. Pancoast tumours may also invade the second and third ribs and also posteriorly into vertebral bodies. They are a rare cause of spinal cord compression if they extend between the intervertebral foramina. Pancoast tumours are often slow to be diagnosed, with initial referral to rheumatologists, physiotherapists and orthopaedic surgeons not uncommon.

- Recurrent laryngeal nerve palsy may also occur as a result of Pancoast tumours but more commonly arise due to lymph node metastases around the left hilum. The left recurrent laryngeal nerve hooks under the arch of the aorta before ascending between the trachea and oesophagus to supply the muscles of the larynx. A left vocal palsy due to lung cancer metastases in the subaortic fossa is more common than a right-sided lesion since the course of the right recurrent laryngeal is comparatively well protected. The CXR often shows a left upper lobe mass or collapsed left upper lobe. A vocal cord palsy causes hoarseness that may be present in 2-18% of lung cancer patients and direct vision at nasendoscopy or bronchoscopy will confirm an adducted, relatively immobile vocal cord. The uncommon scenario of bilateral vocal cord palsies can result in aphonia (an inability to speak) and cause a rapid onset of stridor.

- The phrenic nerve arises from the third, fourth and fifth cervical nerve roots and may be interrupted by lung cancer at any point during its intrathoracic course but commonly in the mediastinum by metastatic lym-phadenopathy. This results in a raised hemidiaphragm and breathlessness, especially in those with underlying COPD, when the dyspnoea can dramati-cally worsen.

- Central tumours may also invade the pericardium, myocardium, pulmonary vasculature and oesophagus. Up to 15% of patients may have cardiac involvement at autopsy, often resulting in pericardial effusion, although tamponade is rare. Pericardial involvement may also cause intractable supraventricular arrhythmias, in particular atrial fibrillation, which may be resistant to antiarrhythmics. Compression of pulmonary vasculature, resulting in mismatch between ventilation and perfusion, is also an important cause of breathlessness in a patient with intrathoracic spread. Limitation of pulmonary blood flow to an area of lung that is adequately ventilated may result in hypoxia. The problem is exacerbated by the fact that many patients with lung cancer have co-existing COPD.

- Dysphagia results from external compression of the middle third of the oesophagus by subcarinal lymphadenopathy or very occasionally by large tracheal tumours. The patient will complain of difficulty swallowing solids initially and then liquids.
- Pleural disease results from direct extension of a peripheral tumour or haematogenous spread. The parietal pleura is equipped with pain fibres that are sensitive to tumour invasion and pleuritic pain (worse on inspiration) may be a particularly debilitating symptom. Pain may difficult to control with standard analgesia and often disrupts quality of life, in particular waking the patient at night. Involvement of the pleura commonly progresses in a pleural effusion, which is another cause of breathlessness in the patient with lung cancer once it becomes large. Approximately 10% of patients have pleural effusions and they may present with an insidious onset of progressive breathlessness over the course of several weeks or months. Characteristic signs of stony dull percussion note, reduced breath sounds over the effusion and reduced vocal resonance will be present.

Symptoms and signs of extrathoracic disease

Patients with lung cancer may also commonly present with symptoms of extrathoracic spread or constitutional symptoms. Lung cancer commonly spreads to supraclavicular lymph nodes, liver, adrenal glands, bones, brain and skin.

- Supraclavicular and anterior cervical nodes may be involved in up to 20% of patients and examination of these areas is vital in the initial assessment of the patient with suspected lung cancer. Aspiration of a lymph node in these regions may reveal crucial diagnostic and staging information.
- Patients with liver involvement may present with severe right upper quadrant pain due to distension of the liver capsule, although this is rare and a late development. This pain is often improved by oral steroid treatment. Metastases may cause obstruction of the hepatic ducts, resulting in raised serum alkaline phosphatase (ALP), raised gamma-glutamyl transferase (γGT) and raised serum bilirubin, manifesting clinically as jaundice. Weight loss is the cardinal symptom of liver involvement and implies a poor prognosis. However, most metastases to liver and adrenals are asymptomatic and are discovered by staging CT scan. Symptoms attributable to adrenal insufficiency are very rare.

- Bone metastases may occur at any site, although the axial skeleton and proximal long bones are most commonly involved. Bone involvement often causes severe pain requiring opiate analgesia and may be present in up to one-fifth of patients at presentation. The ribs are a common site of metastasis and may cause pleuritic pain.
- Metastases to the spinal cord can cause spinal cord compression. This condition can result in severe disability for the patient with lung cancer, so prompt diagnosis, investigations and management are necessary. It is one of the few emergency situations in the presentation of lung cancer. The onset of symptoms is often insidious, with back pain present up to 4 months before spinal cord compression. The recumbent position may worsen pain from vertebral metastasis, in contrast to degenerative joint disease. The emergence of leg weakness, paraesthesias in the lower extremities, and/or bowel or bladder dysfunction should evoke immediate concern for cord compression. Examination may reveal spasticity, hyperreflexia and loss of pinprick, temperature, position and vibratory sensation. Sensation is preserved above a particular dermatome, which is referred to as the sensory level. Percussion tenderness over the affected spinal region may be also present. Deep-tendon reflexes may be initially absent. The Babinski sign (upward movement of the toe in response to plantar stimulation) is also often absent early in the course of compression and lax rectal sphincter tone is a late sign of spinal cord compression. Early recognition of spinal cord compression is the key to preventing permanent sphincter dysfunction. MRI should be the immediate investigation, regardless of normal plain lumbar spine radiographs.
- Lung cancer is the commonest cause of intracranial tumours and of metastases in particular, which are present in up to 10% of patients at presentation. Cerebral involvement most commonly occurs in patients with small-cell lung cancer or adenocarcinoma. Often patients remain asymptomatic initially, but later brain metastases may cause headaches, nausea and vomiting, seizures, hemiplegia, cranial nerve palsies, confusion and changes in personality.

The patient's presenting symptoms of lung cancer may predict prognosis. Patients in whom the diagnosis was made incidentally and who are asymptomatic have the best prognosis. However, patients who present with the constitutional symptoms of anorexia, weight loss and fatigue have been shown to have a higher incidence of metastatic disease (which may be responsible for the symptoms) and therefore a worse prognosis. A standardised evaluation tool for detecting metastatic disease has been proposed by Hooper and colleagues (Table 2.3). The more abnormalities that were found, the higher the likelihood of metastatic disease, although the specific site of metastatic disease would not always be obvious. Clinical assessment of disease spread remains an important initial tool in the assessment of the patient with suspected lung cancer but does not replace sensitive imaging techniques such as CT and in particular positron emission tomography (PET).

Table 2.3 Evaluation of metastatic disease.

Symptoms	Signs	Laboratory tests
Weight loss >10 lb	Lymphadenopathy	Haematocrit <40% in men
Focal skeletal pain	Hoarseness, SVCO	Haematocrit <35% in women
Neurological: headaches, syncope, weakness, confusion	Bone tenderness, hepatomegaly, focal neurological signs, soft-tissue mass	Elevated ALP, γGT

Adapted from Spiro *et al.* (2007).

Paraneoplastic syndromes

The paraneoplastic syndromes are a group of clinical disorders associated with malignant diseases but not physically related to the effects of the primary or secondary tumours. Ten per cent of lung cancer patients have a paraneoplastic syndrome. The severity and extent of the paraneoplastic syndrome is unrelated to the size and stage of the primary tumour. Occasionally, paraneoplastic symptoms may be present before the lung cancer has become apparent, or may signify disease recurrence. The mechanism by which they occur is not entirely understood in all cases, but is often linked to the production of peptides or cytokines by the tumour itself or abnormal host reaction to the tumour (e.g. antibodies). A wide variety of syndromes are associated with lung cancer (see Table 2.4), although those affecting the skeletal, nervous, endocrine and haematological systems are most common.

Musculoskeletal

Digital clubbing is characterised by bulbous uniform swelling of the soft tissue of the terminal phalanx of a digit with subsequent loss of the normal angle between the nail and the nail bed. Several clinical techniques exist for making a diagnosis. Schamroth's test (originally demonstrated by South African cardiologist Dr Leo Schamroth on himself) is a popular test for clubbing. When the distal phalanges of corresponding fingers of opposite hands are directly apposed, a small diamond-shaped 'window' is normally apparent between the nail beds. If this window is obliterated, the test is positive and clubbing is present. The nail profile angle and phalangeal depth ratio can also assist in indentifying clubbing. Hypertrophic pulmonary osteoarthropathy (HPOA) may occur particularly in the context of squamous cell carcinoma of the lung but is associated with all cell types. HPOA is a systemic disorder that involves digital clubbing in addition to a symmetrical arthropathy of wrists and ankles and periosteal new bone formation of the fibula, tibia, radius and ulna. Exceptionally, it can spread to involve the

Table 2.4 Paraneoplastic syndromes associated with lung cancer.

	Common	Rare
General	Anorexia, cachexia, weight loss	Fever, marantic endocarditis
Musculoskeletal	Clubbing, HPOA	
Endocrine	Hypercalcaemia, SIADH	Acromegaly, carcinoid syndrome, hypokalaemic alkalosis, gynaecomastia, lactic acidaemia, hypophosphataemia, hypoglycaemia, hyperthyroidism, elevated LH and FSH
Haematological	Anaemia, polycythaemia	Amyloidosis, leukoerythroblastic reaction, eosinophilia, thrombocytopenia
Neurological	Peripheral neuropathy, LEMS	Mononeuritis multiplex, intestinal pseudo-obstruction, encephalomyelitis, necrotizing myelopathy, cancer-associated retinopathy
Cutaneous	Acanthosis nigricans	Acquired hypertrichosis languinosa, erythema gyratum repens, erythema multiforme, tylosis, erythroderma, exfoliative dermatitis, Sweet syndrome, pruritus, urticaria
Connective tissue	Dermatomyositis	Systemic lupus erythematosus, vasculitis
Renal		Glomerulonephritis, nephrotic syndrome
Coagulopathy	Deep vein thrombosis, pulmonary embolism	Thrombophlebitis, disseminated intravascular coagulation

femur and humerus. The joint surfaces are not involved. Clubbing alone is more common than HPOA and has been described in up to 25% of patients with bronchial carcinoma. The pathogenesis of clubbing and HPOA has not yet been determined. Vascular endothelial growth factor (VEGF) secreted by lung cancer has been implicated. Serum levels of VEGF have been noted to be higher in patients with lung cancer. After resection of the cancer, serum VEGF levels have been noted to fall and analysis of the primary tumour suggested it was the source of ectopic VGEF production. This would support observations that resection of the primary tumour results in regression of clubbing and HPOA.

Endocrine

Lung cancers commonly secrete peptides such as adrenocorticotrophic hormone (ACTH), antidiuretic hormone (ADH), calcitonin, oxytocin and parathyroid hormone-related peptide (PTH-rP). Although elevated levels of these substances may be detected in many patients with lung cancer, only a proportion develop the syndromes with which they are associated.

- A common example of ectopic hormone production is PTH-rP secreted by squamous cell carcinomas, causing hypercalcaemia. Symptoms include polyuria, polydipsia, constipation, abdominal pain, bone pains and confusion. Hypercalcaemia (corrected serum calcium >2.8 mmol/L) causes negative feedback on endogenous PTH production, such that serum PTH levels are characteristically undetectable. PTH-rp released from lung cancer cells results in increased bone resorption, causing hypercalcaemia, in a similar mechanism to endogenous PTH. Hypercalcaemia may also occur in the context of bone metastases alone and should be considered in the differential diagnosis of confusion in the lung cancer patient. Persistent hypercalcaemia that is resistant to intravenous fluid therapy and bisphosphonates represents a poor prognosis.
- Hyponatraemia is a common finding in a patient with lung cancer and may often be due to the syndrome of inappropriate antidiuretic hormone (SIADH). ADH is produced by small-cell lung cancer (which shows neuroendocrine features). It results in an impaired ability to excrete water and may manifest as confusion, seizures and reduced level of consciousness. Biochemically, SIADH is characterised by a serum sodium of less than 135 mmol/L, in the absence of oedema. The serum must be dilute (serum osmolality <260 mmol/kg) and the urine must be inappropriately concentrated (>500 mmol/kg) with continued sodium excretion (urinary sodium concentration >20 mmol/L) to confirm a diagnosis of SIADH. Initiation of cytotoxic chemotherapy for small-cell lung cancer often results in resolution of the syndrome, but subsequent recurrence of hyponatraemia may herald tumour progression.
- Symptoms due to ectopic ACTH production develop in 1% of patients with small-cell carcinoma, but may be more common in pulmonary carcinoid. Patients may occasionally display proximal myopathy, oedema, moon facies, metabolic alkalosis, hypertension and glucose intolerance. Although small-cell lung cancer is responsible for ectopic hormone production in a large number of patients, other endocrine paraneoplastic syndromes are rare.

Neurological

The common neurological paraneoplastic syndromes include peripheral neuropathy, cerebellar degeneration and the Lambert–Eaton myasthenic syndrome. In all of these cases, other neurological illnesses must be excluded before the diagnosis of a paraneoplastic syndrome can be made. Neurological paraneoplastic features are nearly always associated with small-cell carcinomas.

- Peripheral neuropathy may result from an imbalance in vitamin intake and consumption due to the tumour and is common in many malignancies. However, pathological studies have demonstrated inflammatory infiltrates in the areas of the nervous system that correspond to symptoms and have led to the hypothesis that autoantibodies may have a key role. This is supported by the fact that anti-Hu antibodies are nearly always found in the peripheral blood of patients with paraneoplastic neurological syndromes due to lung cancer. Hu antigen is expressed on the surface of small-cell lung cancer and up to 20% of patients will have circulating antibodies, although not all of these patients will demonstrate neurological symptoms and signs. Antibodies are produced by the host's innate immune system in response to previously unrecognised cell surface antigen.
- Patients with Lambert–Eaton myasthenic syndrome (LEMS) experience proximal weakness of the lower limbs that is typically worse in the morning as well as autonomic symptoms such as a dry mouth. It is usually less severe than myasthenia gravis and does not commonly involve the facial muscles or diaphragm. Facilitation (strength improvement after exercise) allows LEMS to be distinguished clinically from myasthenia gravis in which muscles demonstrate fatigability (weakness after exercise). In addition, diplopia, which is characteristic of myasthenia gravis, rarely occurs in LEMS. The syndrome is characterised by IgG antibodies against voltage-gated calcium channels on the presynaptic motor nerve terminal. Although LEMS has been well described in the literature, it remains uncommon, with less than 1% of patients with small-cell lung cancer developing the syndrome. Treatment of the underlying malignancy has yielded variable results in the clinical course of LEMS.

Constitutional symptoms

Anorexia and cachexia of lung cancer are common and may predict the presence of metastatic disease and prognosis. However, these symptoms may be present in patients without distant spread and therefore be considered as a paraneoplastic syndrome. Evidence exists that proteolysis-inducing factor and lipid-mobilising factor are produced by tumour and result in weight loss. Host–tumour interaction results in the excess production of TNFα, IL-1 and IL-6 cytokines, which may also contribute to cachexia. C-Reactive protein is an indirect measure of IL-6 levels and may correlate with symptoms. Anorexia is mediated by the inability of the hypothalamus to respond appropriately to peripheral signals, indicating an energy deficit. Cytokines, including IL-1 and TNFα, appear to mediate this 'hypothalamic resistance'. The cancer cachexia syndrome can have a large impact on quality of life and can lower performance status and outcome.

As with other paraneoplastic syndromes, symptoms may pre-date the discovery of the primary lung cancer. In most cases their occurrence does not reflect stage or prognosis and so it is important that patients should not be precluded from potentially curative therapy on the basis of these syndromes alone.

The history and physical examination of the patient with suspected lung cancer should identify features of the primary as well as metastatic disease and paraneoplastic syndromes and therefore determine the next investigations. In addition, the history should identify risk factors for lung cancer and the patient's performance status, which quantifies patient well-being.

Risk factors for lung cancer

Given that the presenting symptoms of lung cancer are often non-specific, establishing the patient's risk of developing the disease is important in determining which patients to investigate further. Those patients with multiple risk factors for developing lung cancer may warrant investigations even though initial presentation may be unimpressive, for example a dry cough. Smoking is the most important aetiological agent in patients with lung cancer, accounting for 90% of cases in men and 80% in women. The relationship between smoking and lung cancer mortality was first established by Doll and Hill in their cohort study of 40000 medical practitioners and published in 1954 in the *British Medical Journal*. Subsequently, it has been demonstrated that smoking exposure is linearly related to lung cancer risk, so that those patients with a heavy smoking history are at higher risk. It is generally considered that patients with a smoking history of 20 pack years or more are at greatest risk of lung cancer compared with the rest of the population. Chronic obstructive pulmonary disease (COPD) is also usually a consequence of smoking. However, when this important confounding factor is taken into account, COPD has been implicated as an independent risk factor for lung cancer. Therefore patients with airflow limitation are more likely to develop lung cancer than those with normal airway function. Although the vast majority of patients who develop lung cancer (and COPD) have a significant smoking history, the converse is not true. The majority of smokers do not develop lung cancer. Approximately 5% of smokers develop lung cancer, whereas 20% will develop COPD.

Asbestos exposure is a critical risk factor for lung cancer. Some patients may be entitled to compensation, under current UK laws, if lung cancer is thought to be due to asbestos exposure during employment. The precise nature of the exposure and the employment details at the time should be established. Asbestos was formerly used for its remarkable heat-resistant properties and is found in insulation, pipe lagging and brake pads. Lung cancer is estimated to develop in 20-25% of heavily exposed asbestos workers. Smoking has a cumulative effect, further increasing the risk of lung cancer to a factor of 90 versus a factor of 5 in exposed non-smokers. Often, asbestos-related interstitial disease (asbestosis) is associated; however, no correlation exists between the severity of asbestosis and the development of lung cancer. Furthermore, lung cancer has been reported in individuals without interstitial lung disease who are exposed to asbestos. A latency period of 25-35 years is usual. Histologically, the predominant subtype is bronchoalveolar cell carcinoma, but adenocarcinoma and squamous cell carcinoma also occur.

The incidence of lung cancer is also higher in patients who have previously had head and neck malignancy. Other factors that may predispose to bronchogenic lung cancer include pulmonary fibrosis (of any aetiology) and exposure to radon, chromium, arsenic and beryllium. The earliest cases of lung cancer arose in workers exposed to radon in mines in Germany. Patients who have previously had lymphoma treated with thoracic radiotherapy also appear to be at increased risk. A family history of lung cancer has also been implicated in conferring risk up to 2-fold, although no specific genetic defect has been identified.

Performance status

In addition to establishing risk of lung cancer, the history also allows estimation of performance status, which is critical in determining treatment options. Performance status is a function of the patient's overall well-being, which may be affected by patient co-morbidities as well cancer spread. Several scoring systems exist. The Karnofsky score runs from 0 to 100%. The Eastern Co-operative Oncology Group (ECOG) score (Oken *et al*. 1982) is also known as the WHO or Zubrod score and is widely adopted in clinical practice (Table 2.5). The performance status is used to determine whether the patient can receive chemotherapy, whether dose adjustment is necessary, and as a measure for the required intensity of palliative care. It is also used in oncological trials as a measure of quality of life.

In 2005, the National Institute for Clinical Excellence (NICE) first issued guidance on when primary care physicians should consider referral to a lung cancer multidisciplinary team, initially the respiratory physician. Evidence of SVCO or stridor should prompt immediate referral. Patients with persistent haemoptysis or an abnormal CXR should be referred urgently. An urgent CXR may be indicated in patients with haemoptysis, unexplained persistent chest symptoms (>3 weeks), clubbing, lymphadenopathy or features of metastatic spread. Finally, the guidelines point out the importance of the presence of risk factors for lung cancer. Patients who smoke or are ex-smokers, have COPD, or have a history of head and neck cancer and those with asbestos exposure are considered to have a lower threshold for referral for radiography and specialist opinion.

Table 2.5 ECOG score.

Performance status	Description
0	Asymptomatic
1	Symptomatic but completely ambulant
2	Symptomatic, <50% in bed during the day
3	Symptomatic, >50t% in bed but not bedbound
4	Bedbound

Investigation of lung cancer

Investigations will follow the history and examination and are performed with two aims: firstly, to establish the tissue type of lung cancer and, secondly, to accurately demonstrate the extent to which it has spread. These two factors, along with patient physiology and co-morbidity, determine the treatment options. Obtaining a pathological diagnosis distinguishes small-cell and non-small-cell lung cancer. Currently in the UK, a tissue diagnosis is obtained in up to 70% of patients. In a small number of patients who are too frail to undergo investigation other then CXR, a clinical diagnosis alone of lung cancer may be appropriate. In the majority of patients however, a number of investigations are available to make a diagnosis of lung cancer and establish disease stage.

Radiological investigation of lung cancer

Chest radiography

A CXR should be performed in all patients in whom lung cancer is suspected. Lung cancer may present as a solitary pulmonary nodule or mass, pulmonary collapse, pleural effusion or mediastinal lymphadenopathy (see Figs. 2.1 and 2.2). A reliable diagnosis of lung cancer can only be rarely made on CXR and an abnormal CXR is more commonly the trigger for more detailed investigations. The assessment of an abnormality on CXR should always include the examination of previous CXRs where available. In the assessment of a solitary pulmonary nodule, previous CXRs are particularly valuable. It may be possible to ascertain that the nodule has formed at the site of previous infection or infarction or that it has not changed in size over time, making a benign aetiology more likely. If the lesion has not doubled its volume (equivalent to a 26% increase in diameter) over 18 months, it is highly unlikely to be malignant. However, if the lesion increases in size very rapidly, infection and infarction become more likely possibilities.

Where a CXR has been requested in primary or secondary care and is suggestive of lung cancer, a copy of the radiologist's report in most institutions is sent to the thoracic physician member of the lung multidisciplinary team for follow-up. Although few published data are available on the sensitivity and specificity of CXR in lung cancer, it is important to recognise that the CXR remains an insensitive tool. Therefore, if lung cancer is suspected clinically and the CXR is negative, the patient should still be referred to the thoracic physician.

Computed tomography

Computed tomography (CT) scanning provides cross-sectional imaging and is invaluable for the diagnosis and staging of lung cancer. It allows detailed anatomical information to be obtained about the primary lesion and also offers an indication of metastatic spread to the mediastinum and extrathoracic structures. CT should be performed in all patients in whom treatment (radical or palliative) is being considered. In addition to the thorax, imaging of the liver

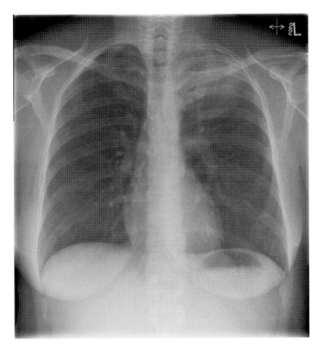

Fig. 2.1 Chest radiograph (CXR) showing right-sided lung mass. Percutaneous biopsy under CT guidance demonstrated this to be a well-differentiated lung adenocarcinoma.

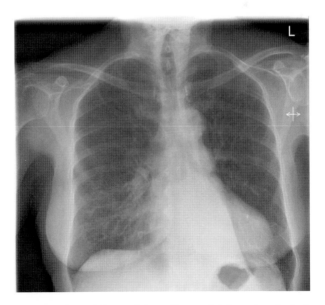

Fig. 2.2 CXR showing left lower lobe collapse. A triangular shaped opacity is seen behind the cardiac shadow and the left hemidiaphragm is obscured medially. Bronchoscopy revealed squamous cell carcinoma obstructing the left lower lobe orifice.

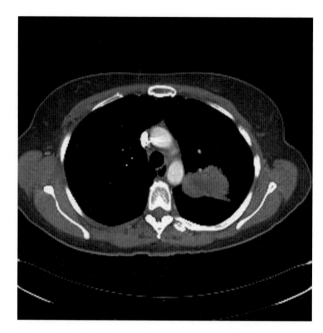

Fig. 2.3 CT scan showing heterogeneous peripheral lung mass. Percutaneous biopsy revealed adenocarcinoma.

and adrenals (to which lung cancer commonly spreads) is included and use of intravenous contrast medium allows discrimination of vascular structures. CT accurately locates the primary lesion (which guides the best biopsy approach) and also provides morphological information that may predict the probability of malignancy of a pulmonary nodule. Nodules with diffuse calcification have been reliably shown to be benign. Several features of pulmonary nodules may be combined to give up to 90% sensitivity of detecting malignancy. These features include the presence of spicules, inhomogeneity, areas of necrosis, evidence of local or vascular invasion and ground-glass opacity of lung parenchyma adjacent to the lesion. The low specificity, however, means that lesions should be biopsied in all cases before a diagnosis of lung cancer is confirmed (Fig. 2.3).

CT is often unable to demonstrate chest wall or direct mediastinal invasion with sufficient accuracy. Particularly in the case of mediastinal invasion, this may affect whether the patient is a candidate for curative surgery or not. In these cases magnetic resonance imaging (MRI) has an important role. Another disadvantage of CT is in assessment of the mediastinum. By convention, mediastinal nodes less than 1 cm in the short axis are considered to be benign. However, several studies have demonstrated malignancy in mediastinal lymph nodes of less than 1 cm. Therefore, CT has a low sensitivity of 50% for detecting mediastinal spread. Twenty per cent of mediastinal nodes that are normal by CT criteria (<1 cm) may contain malignant disease. Additionally, specificity for mediastinal spread is also low. CT may detect enlarged mediastinal nodes that are not due to malignant spread and up to 40% of enlarged mediastinal nodes are benign. These problems highlight the importance of obtaining a tissue diagnosis when considering mediastinal metastases.

CT has a far superior sensitivity for detecting extrathoracic spread of lung cancer. It may demonstrate the presence of asymptomatic supraclavicular lymphadenopathy or bone or liver metastases and therefore identify extrathoracic disease amenable to biopsy, providing crucial diagnostic and staging information. CT of the brain is not usually carried out routinely in the absence of neurological symptoms or signs. In patients with intrathoracic disease only, CT identifies proximal lesions that are amenable to biopsy by bronchoscopy and more peripheral lesions that may be better suited to per-cutaneous radiology guided biopsy. CT can therefore improve the accuracy of the first invasive investigation. By performing CT as a first test, bronchoscopy may be prevented in up to 17% of cases by demonstrating that the lesion is too peripheral for bronchoscopy or that extrathoracic disease is present that could be biopsied. CT should therefore always be carried out before bron-choscopy and is considered an essential procedure for most patients with suspected lung cancer.

Ultrasonography

Ultrasound imaging of the neck has a role in patients with lung cancer and suspected mediastinal metastases. One study has suggested a high preva-lence of impalpable malignant supraclavicular nodes in patients with enlarged mediastinal nodes on CT. Ultrasound-guided fine-needle aspiration (FNA) of malignant supraclavicular nodes provides a cytological diagnosis and sufficient staging information to guide treatment options. Some centres therefore routinely include ultrasound scanning of the neck in the diagnostic and staging algorithm for lung cancer. Ultrasound is also useful for distin-guishing between benign cysts and metastases in the liver and may be used to guide peripheral lung biopsies in some cases.

Magnetic resonance imaging

Magnetic resonance imaging (MRI) is superior to CT in the evaluation of superior sulcus tumours as well as for determining chest wall or mediastinal invasion. There are no recent studies on the use of MRI in the assessment of the mediastinum; however, given the evolution of newer technologies in MRI this area warrants further investigation. MRI is an established first-line test for the detection of spinal cord metastases and should be performed urgently in patients with suspected spinal cord compression.

Radionuclide bone scanning

Radionuclide bone scanning is a sensitive test for detecting bone metastases. Intravenous injection of a radionuclide (commonly technetium-99m) is followed 2-3 hours later by scanning with a gamma camera that is sensitive to the radiation emitted by the injected material. False-positive results may occur owing to arthritis, infection or trauma, and therefore bone scan is not routinely undertaken without clinical suspicion. A solitary lesion should be further evaluated with plain radiograph or MRI before being labelled as metastatic disease. Multiple areas of abnormality are more highly suggestive of metastatic disease. Bone scan is also occasionally associated with false-negative results, particularly with lytic lesions due to adenocarcinoma.

Positron emission tomography

Positron emission tomography (PET) scanning is performed after the administration of [^{18}F]fluorodeoxyglucose (FDG), which is a glucose analogue that has been tagged with the positron-emitting isotope fluorine-18. Patients are asked to fast for 6 hours prior to the scan. Malignant cells have a higher glucose metabolism than normal tissue and so take up more FDG than the surrounding tissue and emit a greater number of positrons. The standardised uptake value (SUV), the measure of metabolic activity detected by PET, is directly related to the degree of metabolic activity within a tissue focus and provides predictive information regarding treatment response and survival. An SUV of 2.5 is regarded as the upper limit of normal in an attempt to minimise the chance of false-negative results. However, false-negative results still occur in tumours with low metabolic activity such as adenocarcinoma, bronchoalveolar carcinoma and carcinoid tumours. PET scans may also be falsely positive due to granulomatous conditions and other inflammatory disorders, including infections. The spatial resolution of current PET scanners is limited to 7–8 mm and the use of PET to characterise solitary pulmonary nodules is restricted to lesions of >1 cm, although the metabolic activity of the tumour is likely to be major determinant rather than size alone.

PET scanning is recommended by NICE in all non-small-cell lung cancer (NSCLC) patients in whom curative treatment is proposed. PET is cost-effective and has high accuracy for overall disease staging in patients with NSCLC (Table 2.6). PET scanning may have a superior sensitivity to bone scanning for detecting bone metastases and overall may detect distant disease in 20% of patients who were previously being considered for surgical cure. Recently, fusion PET-CT imaging has become more widely available and represents an advance on PET alone with better spatial resolution and superior accuracy and sensitivities for disease staging (Fig. 2.4).

PET scanning can also provide important information to assist in radiotherapy treatment planning and in guiding biopsy of a primary or metastatic lesion. Despite its advantages over CT in the systemic staging of NSCLC, PET has distinct limitations as a screening tool for mediastinal metastasis. The negative predictive value of PET is generally considered to be excellent at over 97%. However, the sensitivity for detecting tumour metastasis varies depending on the lymph node's location within the mediastinum. Although PET has excellent sensitivity (80–99%) in detecting metastasis to paratracheal and hilar nodes, its sensitivity at other mediastinal lymph node stations (e.g. subcarinal) is unsatisfactory (29–60%). In addition to a high false-negative rate with screening for metastases at certain mediastinal lymph

Table 2.6 Performance characteristics of CT, PET and PET-CT for staging of NSCLC.

	Accuracy (%)	Specificity (%)	Sensitivity (%)	PPV (%)	NPV (%)
General disease staging					
PET	80	71	100	63	100
PET-CT	84	76	100	67	100
Mediastinal staging					
CT	56–75	71	50	31–60	74–80
PET	78–82	79	67–94	49	98

PPV: positive predictive value. NPV: negative predictive value.

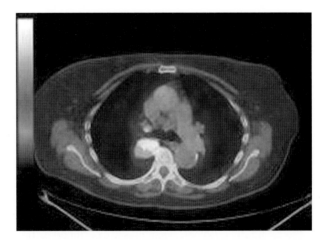

Fig. 2.4 Fusion PET-CT showing FDG-avid peripheral right sided lung mass and subcarinal mediastinal node. Sampling of the subcarinal node revealed it to be benign and the patient underwent curative surgery.

node stations, false-positive results also occur. Up to 25% of FDG-avid positive mediastinal lesions are due to benign conditions. Patients should therefore not be denied curative surgery on the basis of FDG-avid mediastinal disease alone and tissue confirmation is necessary (see Fig. 2.4). In specific cases where enlarged mediastinal nodes are present on CT and the PET scan is negative, pathological confirmation may still be required. Patients with no mediastinal disease on the basis of CT and PET have a low likelihood of mediastinal metastasis. Therefore, in general, treatment decisions should not be based on PET scan alone and results should be interpreted in the light of location and size of mediastinal disease.

Although FDG is the most widely utilised PET metabolite, [¹¹C]choline is emerging as a potential superior alternative. Choline is taken up by cells via a transmembrane transport protein that is increased in tumour cells. Increased

[^{11}C]choline activity is therefore indicative of tumour proliferation. Choline-PET has been shown to have greater sensitivity (100%) than FDG-PET (75%) in a prospective trial of 29 patients who underwent FDG-PET as well as [^{11}C]choline-PET followed by surgical resection and mediastinal lymph node dissection (Hara *et al.* 2000). Additional studies are required to validate its clinical use.

Investigations for tissue confirmation of lung cancer

Sputum cytology

Sputum cytology is a non-invasive method of diagnosing lung cancer by detecting exfoliated malignant cells. Sensitivity is higher for central squamous cell and small-cell carcinomas than for more peripheral adenocarcinomas and in order to increase yield a minimum of three samples should be collected. A positive finding for malignancy from a cytological specimen is accurate in up to 90% of cases and is a rapid and inexpensive investigation. However, distinction between different subtypes of lung cancer is often not possible and discordant results have been observed between sputum cytology and histological findings from bronchoscopy. Abnormal cells may result from anywhere in the aerodigestive tract and also from preinvasive lesions that may be difficult to locate with conventional bronchoscopy. In view of these disadvantages, sputum cytology as a sole test is confined to patients who are unwilling or unable to tolerate bronchoscopy or transthoracic biopsy.

Bronchoscopy

Bronchoscopy allows tissue confirmation of lung cancer and has a sensitivity of 80% for centrally located lesions. The procedure is performed on an outpatient basis under conscious sedation and may be approached via the nose or mouth. Cytological samples are obtained by bronchial brushings and washings, but the highest yield and accuracy are provided by biopsy of a visible endobronchial lesion. The incidence of serious complications is extremely low and bronchoscopy is regarded as a standard procedure for the diagnosis of central lesions. In addition to providing pathological information, bronchoscopy also allows assessment of the location and extent of the endobronchial lesion (which may impact significantly on treatment), while demonstration of a paralysed vocal cord implies mediastinal invasion and inoperability.

The advent of autofluorescence bronchoscopy, which uses blue light rather than the standard white-light bronchoscopy, allows identification of preinvasive lesions that may be missed by usual techniques. Observations in the lung have shown that dysplasia, carcinoma in situ, and microinvasive carcinomas exhibit weaker green fluorescence than normal tissues when illuminated with blue light. Normal endobronchial mucosa therefore appears green, while the abnormal areas appear red. The natural history of these preinvasive lesions remains unclear, however, with some regressing while others progress to frankly invasive disease, and so the role of autofluorescence bronchoscopy in clinical practice remains to be identified.

Transthoracic needle aspiration

Transthoracic needle aspiration or biopsy is the investigation of choice for patients with peripheral lung lesions. It involves the insertion of a needle percutaneously, under conscious sedation, to sample tissue from the lung that is then examined for malignancy. CT, ultrasound or fluoroscopy is used to guide needle insertion. Fine-needle aspiration (20-22 gauge) provides material for cytology, whereas larger-diameter needles (16-18 gauge) can provide tissue cores for histology. Sensitivity of the procedure is over 80%, although a biopsy that is negative for malignancy may warrant further investigations if the clinical suspicion remains high. The most common complication is pneumothorax, which may occur in up to 30% of procedures, requiring a chest drain in 5-10% of cases. A pneumothorax is more likely to occur if the patient has evidence of emphysema on the CT scan and some centres will not carry out the investigation if the FEV_1 is less than 1 litre, since a pneumothorax would be poorly tolerated in these patients. Other factors that predict pneumothorax include the size of the lesion and the distance in the lung through which the needle must traverse in order to reach the lesion. Lesions that are smaller and that are farther from the lung edge have a higher risk of pneumothorax. Other complications of transthoracic biopsy include haemorrhage and tumour seeding the needle track, but these are very rare.

Mediastinoscopy

Mediastinoscopy or mediastinotomy may be required for central tumours that are extraluminal and therefore inaccessible by standard bronchoscopy. Further investigation of the mediastinum may also be required in patients who otherwise may have operable lung cancer. Standard cervical mediastinoscopy affords access to the upper and lower paratracheal regions anteriorly and the upper subcarinal nodes (see Fig. 2.6). Nodes on the left and in particular the aortopulmonary window are best accessed via left anterior mediastinotomy. These surgical procedures require general anaesthesia and typically an in-patient overnight stay. However, they do allow large histological specimens to be obtained and, importantly, microscopic malignant disease can be identified. Complications of bleeding, pain and infection are uncommon and mortality is very rare. Because mediastinoscopy is able to sample only some of the lymph node stations, its sensitivity for detecting mediastinal spread from lung cancer is 80%.

Endobronchial and endoscopic ultrasound

Endobronchial and endoscopic ultrasound-guided fine-needle aspiration are newer techniques that allow minimally invasive sampling of the mediastinum and provide diagnostic and staging information (Fig. 2.5). Both procedures are safely carried out in outpatients under conscious sedation. Endobronchial ultrasound (EBUS) combines standard bronchoscopy with an ultrasound probe at the tip in addition to the conventional white light. Once contact is made with the tracheobronchial wall (by inflating a balloon around the ultrasound probe), mediastinal structures are visible by ultrasound and can be

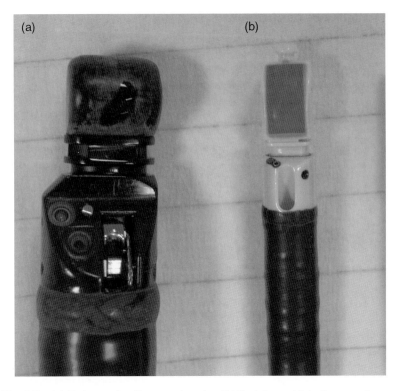

Fig. 2.5 (a) Endoscopic ultrasound probe. (b) Endobronchial ultrasound probe. Both probes allow minimally invasive sampling of mediastinal lymph nodes and masses.

sampled under direct vision with high sensitivity and specificity. EBUS is able to visualise parabronchial masses and lymph nodes at stations 2, 3, 4, 5, 7 and 10 (see Fig. 2.6). Endoscopic ultrasound (EUS) is a complementary procedure to EBUS. A gastroscope with an ultrasound processor at the tip is placed in the oesophagus at approximately 35–30 cm from the mouth. The location of the oesophagus makes EUS most effective for left-sided lesions and affords access to lymph node stations 3, 4L, 5, 7, 8 and 9. The combination of EBUS and EUS therefore allows minimally invasive sampling of almost all mediastinal lymph nodes and far more than mediastinoscopy alone. EBUS and EUS together have a sensitivity of over 90% for detecting mediastinal spread from lung cancer.

Video-assisted thorascopic surgery

Thoracotomy or video-assisted thorascopic surgery (VATS) may be necessary in rare cases when other less-invasive techniques have failed to determine the diagnosis. Both procedures allow direct visualisation of the lesion by the thoracic surgeon under general anaesthesia. Thoracotomy is usually performed via the posterolateral approach. An incision is made between the ribs and the ribs are held apart, allowing the surgeon access to any area of the lung or mediastinum. Thoracotomy is a major undertaking and is therefore usually reserved for cases

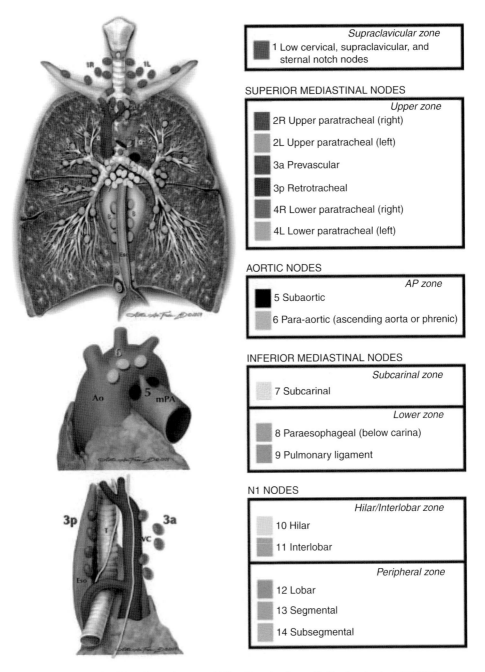

Fig. 2.6 Mediastinal lymph node map. (After Dresler from Detterbeck *et al.* (2009); reproduced with kind permission of ACCP.)

where the lung cancer may be resected with curative intent. The lesion may be biopsied initially and an on-site pathologist can provide confirmation of malignancy by assessment of a 'frozen section' sample. VATS biopsy is far less invasive but does not usually allow effective curative surgery to be carried out at the same time. It is analogous to abdominal laparoscopic surgery and involves the insertion of a camera (videothorascope) and biopsy forceps via small incisions. The procedure allows access to all areas within the thorax and therefore has a high sensitivity for diagnosing (and staging) lung cancer.

Investigation of pleural effusions

Pleural effusions are a presenting feature in 10% of patients with lung cancer. Pleural aspiration should always be the first test; diagnostic yield in a malignant effusion is high (70%) and may be increased by obtaining three separate samples of at least 20 mL. CT or ultrasound guided pleural biopsy should be obtained if aspiration is negative and is more effective than blind pleural biopsy with an Abram's needle. Thoracoscopy (medical or video-assisted thoracic surgery, VATS) is more invasive but allows direct visualisation of the pleural cavity and biopsy of the parietal pleura, providing a diagnosis in up to 95% of cases of malignant pleural effusion. Thoracoscopy also provides an opportunity to proceed directly to talc pleurodesis. Medical thoracoscopy is carried out in some centres under local anaesthesia and conscious sedation only.

Staging of lung cancer

Once a diagnosis of lung cancer has been made, attention turns to determining the extent to which the disease has spread. Staging provides a guide to treatment options and prognosis. An internationally agreed staging definition also allows patient groups to be accurately compared. Staging may be based on clinical grounds or on findings from surgical pathology specimens.

Non-small-cell carcinoma

Non-small-cell lung cancer (NSCLC) is staged according to the T (tumour) N (node) M (metastasis) system. The system was derived from a database of over 5000 patients treated for NSCLC from 1975 to 1988. It has since been updated and was reviewed in 2009. The current TNM definitions are summarised in Table 2.7 and the effect of lung cancer on survival is demonstrated in Table 2.8. Patients presenting at earlier stages of NSCLC have a better prognosis with 5-year survival for stage I disease at over 55%. Unfortunately, the majority of patients present with metastatic disease and 5-year survival for stage IV NSCLC is only 1%. Distinguishing between hilar and mediastinal disease is critical for treatment options. Patients who have disease confined to hilar lymph glands are considered candidates for curative therapy (stage II and stage IIIA-N1). Hilar glands are regarded as being located within the visceral pleura. The presence of mediastinal disease (as defined by lymphadenopathy within the mediastinal pleural reflection) implies stage III disease and usually confers inoperability although controversy remains on how to best manage patients with stage IIIA-N2 disease (see Chapter 3).

Table 2.7 TNM definitions in non-small-cell lung cancer.

Descriptors	Definitions	Subgroups*
T	**Primary tumour**	
T0	No primary tumour	
T1	Tumour ≤3 cm[†], surrounded by lung or visceral pleura, not more proximal than the lobar bronchus	
T1a	Tumour ≤2 cm[†]	T1a
T1b	Tumour >2 but ≤3 cm[†]	T1b
T2	Tumour >3 but ≤7 cm[†] or tumour with any of the following[‡]: Invades visceral pleura, involves main bronchus ≥2 cm distal to the carina, atelectasis/ obstructive pneumonia extending to hilum but not involving the entire lung	
T2a	Tumour >3 but ≤5 cm[†]	T2a
T2b	Tumour >5 but ≤7 cm[†]	T2b
T3	Tumour >7 cm	T3$_{>7}$
	or directly invading chest wall, diaphragm, phrenic nerve, mediastinal pleura, or parietal pericardium	T3$_{Inv}$
	or tumour in the main bronchus <2 cm distal to the carina[§]	T3$_{Centr}$
	or atelectasis/obstructive pneumonitis of entire lung	T3$_{Centr}$
	or separate tumour nodules in the same lobe	T3$_{Satell}$
T4	Tumour of any size with invasion of heart, great vessels, trachea, recurrent laryngeal nerve, oesophagus, vertebral body, or carina	T4$_{Inv}$
	or separate tumour nodules in a different ipsilateral lobe	T4$_{Ipsi Nod}$
N	**Regional lymph nodes**	
N0	No regional node metastasis	
N1	Metastasis in ipsilateral peribronchial and/or perihilar lymph nodes and intrapulmonary nodes, including involvement by direct extension	
N2	Metastasis in ipsilateral mediastinal and/or subcarinal lymph nodes	
N3	Metastasis in contralateral mediastinal, contralateral hilar, ipsilateral or contralateral scalene, or supraclavicular lymph nodes	
M	**Distant metastasis**	
M0	No distant metastasis	
M1a	Separate tumour nodules in a contralateral lobe	M1a$_{Contr Nod}$
	or tumour with pleural nodules or malignant pleural dissemination[‖]	M1a$_{Pl Dissem}$
M1b	Distant metastasis	M1b
		(*Continued*)

Table 2.7 (*Continued*)

Descriptors	Definitions	Subgroups*
Special situations		
TX, NX, MX	T, N, or M status not able to be assessed	
Tis	Focus of in situ cancer	Tis
T1§	Superficial spreading tumour of any size but confined to the wall of the trachea or mainstem bronchus	T1$_{ss}$

Definitions for T, N, M Descriptors from Detterbeck *et al.* (2009) reproduced with permission.
*These subgroup labels are not defined in the IASLC publications but are added here to facilitate a clear discussion.
†In the greatest dimension.
‡T2 tumours with these features are classified as T2a if ≤5 cm.
§The uncommon superficial spreading tumour in central airways is classified as T1.
‖Pleural effusions are excluded that are cytologically negative, non-bloody, transudative, and clinically judged not to be due to cancer.

Table 2.8 Non-small-cell lung cancer staging and survival.

Stage	TNM	Percentage surviving 5 years
0	Carcinoma in situ	
IA	T1 N0 M0	65–70
IB	T2 N0 M0	55–60
IIA	T1 N1 M0	50–55
IIB	T2 N1 M0	35–40
	T3 N0 M0	30–35
IIIA	T3 N1 M0	20–25
	T1 N2 M0	15–20
	T2 N2 M0	
	T3 N2 M0	
IIIB	T4 N0 M0	5–10
	T4 N1 M0	
	T4 N2 M0	
	T1 N3 M0	3–5
	T2 N3 M0	
	T3 N3 M0	
	T4 N3 M0	
IV	Any T, Any N, M1	1

After Detterbeck *et al.* (2007).

Small-cell carcinoma

Small-cell lung cancer grows rapidly and there is usually evidence of extrapulmonary disease at presentation. The Veterans Administration Lung Cancer Study Group (VALG) introduced 'limited' and 'extensive' disease and this has been adopted in clinical practice. The TNM system was thought to have limited use for small-cell lung cancer except in rare patients who are to undergo surgical resection. Historically, limited disease refers to small-cell lung cancer confined to the ipsilateral hemithorax and supraclavicular lymph nodes only. Two-thirds of patients present with evidence of metastatic spread and are staged as extensive disease. Recent research, however, recommends TNM staging of small-cell lung cancer. A large epidemiological study found that survival was directly related to both T and N categories. Differences were more pronounced in patients without mediastinal or supraclavicular nodal involvement. Stage grouping of TNM also demonstrates differences in survival except between IA and IB. Patients with pleural effusion regardless of the cytology have an intermediate prognosis between limited and extensive disease (Shepherd *et al.* 2007).

An algorithm for the diagnosis and staging of non-small-cell lung cancer

Patients with lung cancer should be diagnosed and staged to the highest level using as few tests as possible. However, the staging of lung cancer is necessarily complex and often involves several procedures after history and physical examination. The aim remains to obtain a tissue diagnosis and then accurately establish disease stage to guide treatment and prognosis.

Patients who have extrathoracic disease amenable to biopsy (e.g. liver metastases) should have this area sampled as a first investigation, thereby providing a tissue diagnosis and disease stage in a single test. Similarly, patients with pleural effusion should have this investigated, as a positive result of malignancy will distinguish small-cell lung cancer and non-small-cell lung cancer and stage the patient as having IIIB disease in the case of NSCLC.

In NSCLC, determining whether there are metastases to mediastinal nodes is of paramount importance. Diagnosing mediastinal spread in the otherwise operable patient may have the catastrophic consequence of missing an opportunity to operate. Conversely, and more commonly, missing mediastinal metastases may mean the patient undergoes a thoracotomy and lung resection for no benefit. An algorithm taking into account the sensitivities and specificities of investigations in NSCLC discussed above is presented in Figure 2.7. Patients with intrathoracic disease only should have tissue confirmation of the mediastinum before surgery is performed except in cases where both CT and PET suggest the mediastinum is negative for metastatic disease. However, in case of central tumours, PET-positive hilar N1 disease, low FDG uptake of the primary tumour and lymph nodes ≥10 mm on CT scan, invasive mediastinal staging remains indicated. Surgery should not be precluded in patients with CT-or PET-positive mediastinal nodes without pathological confirmation. Improving the selection of patients who are suitable for radical treatment is an area of ongoing research.

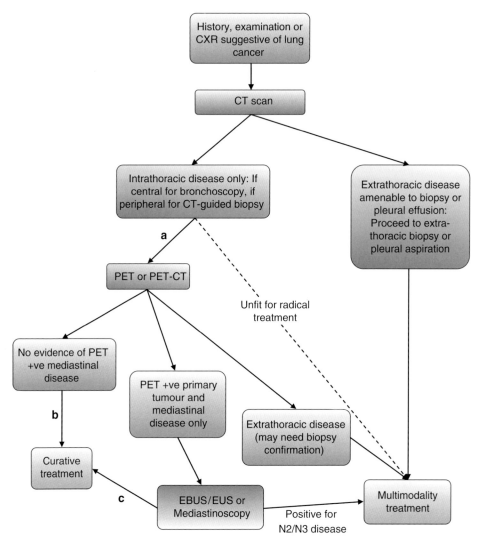

Fig. 2.7 Algorithm for the diagnosis and staging of non-small-cell lung cancer.
a: Candidate for radical treatment. b: Invasive mediastinal staging is still required if the tumour is central, there is PET-positive hilar N1 disease, low FDG uptake of the primary tumor or lymph nodes ≥10 mm on CT scan. c: EBUS or EUS may be the first invasive test for mediastinal staging, but if negative should be followed by surgical staging before radical treatment is offered.

Mesothelioma

Mesothelioma is a malignant disease of serosal surfaces, such as the pleura and peritoneum, and is closely associated with previous asbestos exposure. The incidence of mesothelioma is rapidly increasing and in the UK the burden of disease is likely to peak between 2011 and 2015 with approximately 2000 deaths per year.

The clinical features of mesothelioma

Unlike lung cancer, mesothelioma rarely presents with symptoms of meta-static spread or paraneoplastic syndromes. Eighty per cent of cases occur in men and the earliest symptoms are usually chest pain or breathlessness. The pain is usually dull, occasionally worse on inspiration, and progresses inexora-bly during the course of the illness. In some cases the tumour invades inter-costal nerves, resulting in a neuropathic pain that may be resistant to usual analgesia. Breathlessness is usually due to a pleural effusion, but later in the disease course may result from the restrictive effects of pleural thickening. Weight loss and fatigue occur in less than 30% of patients at presentation but are universally present as the illness progresses. Mesothelioma may also pre-sent with a chest wall mass or rarely with a pneumothorax. Peritoneal involve-ment may cause ascites, abdominal pain and bowel obstruction. In addition to the pleura and peritoneum, mesothelioma may develop on other serosal sur-faces, such as the pericardium and tunica vaginalis, although the pleura is by far the most common site.

Physical examination may reveal signs consistent with a pleural effusion or ascites. Advanced pleural thickening results in reduced expansion on the affected side. Clubbing occurs in less than 1% of cases. Subcutaneous masses are relatively uncommon at presentation and usually suggest prior medical intervention and occur in drainage sites and thoracotomy scars.

Local invasion of the tumour is more common than haematogenous spread. Direct involvement of mediastinal structures is common, but hoarseness and superior vena caval obstruction are rare clinical features. Distant metastases rarely cause symptoms at presentation, although they are often present at postmortem. The contralateral lung is invaded by pleural mesothelioma in 10-20% of cases. Constitutional symptoms, such as weight loss and fatigue generally appear late in the disease course and indicate a poor prognosis.

Asbestos exposure

Over 85% of cases of mesothelioma are directly attributable to occupational asbestos exposure and mesothelioma was rare before the widespread use of asbestos. Evidence of the association between asbestos and mesothelioma was first published in 1960 from data in South Africa.

There are two forms of asbestos: long, thin fibres known as amphiboles (one type of which is called blue asbestos) and feathery fibres known as chrysotile or white asbestos. Both forms are thought to be carcinogenic, but the higher rate of mesothelioma is seen with amphibole exposure. The mechanism by which asbestos fibres cause mesothelioma is not fully understood. One pos-sibility is that the asbestos fibres protrude from the lung surface and cause repeated cycles of scratching, damage, inflammation and repair eventually resulting in malignant transformation. This is supported by the observation that mesotheliomas occur initially in the parietal mesothelium rather than on the visceral surface.

The latency period between first exposure to asbestos and development of mesothelioma is typically very long. Very few cases occur with less than 20 years latency and nearly a third arise after 40 years.

The highest mesothelioma risks tend to be in those patients who have worked in shipbuilding, railway engineering and construction, where they experienced high levels of asbestos exposure. Para-occupational exposure, particularly in women who have washed their husband's clothes, may also cause mesothelioma and must be included in a detailed occupational history. Measurements of airborne asbestos levels in buildings containing asbestos are several orders of magnitude lower than levels to which asbestos workers are exposed and are unlikely to result in malignant mesothelioma. The history of asbestos exposure is very important but is often not recalled by the patient at presentation.

Many workers have been exposed to asbestos and will be aware of the potential health consequences. However, only a minority of patients go onto to develop life-threatening disease. Unfortunately, there is currently no evidence to suggest that screening exposed individuals is of any benefit.

Referral

Referral for specialist opinion should be considered in all cases of an unexplained pleural effusion or pleural thickening, particularly in the context of chest pain, breathlessness or asbestos exposure.

Investigations

Investigations aim to provide an accurate and rapid diagnosis, which is important for therapeutic, prognostic and medico-legal reasons. The most frequent dilemma is the differentiation of mesothelioma from metastatic adenocarcinoma involving the pleura. Both conditions tend to arise in elderly men and often present with chest pain, breathlessness and pleural effusion. Additionally, first-line investigations may fail to yield a diagnosis of mesothelioma, although the clinical suspicion remains high. This scenario is not uncommon and clinical follow-up is warranted.

Imaging

Chest radiography is the most common initial investigation. It often demonstrates a unilateral pleural effusion or pleural thickening and should prompt further investigations. In patients with very advanced tumour, an encasing rind of tumour may be evident.

CT scanning often shows only a pleural effusion but may in some cases also demonstrate pleural thickening. Irregular thickening of the mediastinal pleural surface may indicate a higher likelihood of malignant disease. CT commonly also indicates evidence of asbestos exposure. Calcified pleural plaques are most commonly found along the diaphragm and are usually demonstrated on CXR as well. They should be regarded as markers of asbestos exposure only and should not be considered as precursors to malignancy. Rounded atelectasis, or folded lung, is a benign pleurally-based mass lesion associated with asbestos that can mimic mesothelioma or lung cancer. It forms as a result of local inflammation that results in a portion of the lung becoming adherent to the pleura. As well as demonstrating intrathoracic spread from mesothelioma, CT can also show extrathoracic disease.

MRI has a role in cases where it is important to identify invasion into the chest wall or diaphragm. PET should be performed in the rare cases when surgical cure is proposed. It has a high sensitivity for detecting lymph node and extrathoracic disease.

Cytopathology

If imaging confirms a pleural effusion, pleural aspiration should be the next investigation. Blood-stained fluid is often obtained and should be sent to the cytology laboratory to be centrifuged and a cell block prepared. Although malignancy is diagnosed with confidence on cytological specimens, it is not always possible to distinguish mesothelioma from metastatic adenocarcinoma. In these cases, a biopsy sample of tumour tissue is usually taken for histopathological analysis.

Histopathology

Biopsy samples of thickened pleura should be obtained with a cutting needle under direct radiological guidance. This technique has a higher sensitivity than blind bedside biopsy with an Abram's needle, which is positive in only 30–50% of cases of mesothelioma. Medical thoracoscopy and VATS provide the best means for pleural biopsy under direct vision and also allow pleurodesis at the same procedure. However, since adenocarcinoma may resemble mesothelioma macroscopically and microscopically, biopsy in some cases may be unhelpful and immunohistochemistry has an important role.

Immunohistochemistry can determine that the tissue is of mesothelial origin (calretinin positive) and that it is malignant mesothelioma (epithelial membrane antigen positive). Cytokeratin stains are important for confirming invasion and distinguishing mesothelioma from sarcomas and melanoma. CEA and TTF-1 are almost never expressed in mesothelioma, whereas positive staining for calretinin and epithelial membrane antigen suggest mesothelioma. Where results are equivocal by immunohistochemistry, electron microscopy helps distinguish mesothelioma from adenocarcinoma.

Blood tests

Non-specific features of malignancy may manifest in the blood tests, for example raised ESR, anaemia and low albumin. Some centres use serum mesothelin-related protein (SMRP) as an adjunct for mesothelioma diagnosis.

SMRP is the circulating product of mesothelin, a surface protein thought to be important in mesothelial cell adhesion. In one study, 84% of patients with mesothelioma had elevated concentrations of SMRP, compared with less than 2% of patients with other pleural or malignant processes. Levels may also parallel disease progression. Recent evidence also suggests SMRP may also be found in pleural effusions of patients with mesothelioma. Its role in screening asbestos-exposed individuals for mesothelioma is an area of future research.

Pulmonary function tests

Encasement of the lung by malignant mesothelioma results in a restrictive pattern and increased expiratory flow rates. Lung volumes may be directly influenced by the amount of pleural fluid. However, if there is no change to the amount of pleural fluid, changes in forced vital capacity (FVC) are an accurate guide to disease progression.

Staging

TNM staging is rarely employed in the management of mesothelioma, except in rare instances of surgical resection. The International Mesothelioma Interest Group developed a staging system based on lung cancer staging that also reflects prognosis. Accurate preoperative assessment requires definitive tissue diagnosis and assessment with CT and PET scan and possibly MRI and mediastinoscopy. Often, definitive staging is only possible at surgery.

Summary

Lung cancer is the commonest cause of cancer death and smoking is the main aetiological factor in its pathogenesis. Symptoms occur late in the natural history of lung cancer and therefore the majority of lung cancers present late with advanced disease. Presenting symptoms and signs may suggest the location and extent of lung cancer. Investigations allow accurate diagnosis and staging and are essential to guide treatment and prognosis.

References

Detterbeck, F.C., Jantz, M.A., Wallace, M., Vansteenkiste, J. and Silvestri, G.A. (2007) American College of Chest Physicians. Invasive mediastinal staging of lung cancer: ACCP evidence-based clinical practice guidelines (2nd edition). *Chest*, **132** (3 Suppl.), 202S-220S.

Geddes, D.M. (1979) The natural history of lung cancer: a review based on rates of tumour growth. *British Journal of Diseases of the Chest*, **73** (1), 1-17.

Hara, T., Inagaki, K., Kosaka, N. and Morita, T. (2000) Sensitive detection of mediastinal lymph node metastasis of lung cancer with ^{11}C-choline PET. *Journal of Nuclear Medicine*, **41**, 1507-1513.

Oken, M.M., Creech, R.H., Tormey, D.C., *et al.* (1982) Toxicity and response criteria of the Eastern Cooperative Oncology Group. *American Journal of Clinical Oncology*, **5** (6), 649–655.

Shepherd, F., Crowley, J., Van Houtte, P., *et al.* (2007) The International Association for the Study of Lung Cancer Lung Cancer Staging Project: Proposals regarding the clinical staging of small-cell lung cancer in the forthcoming (seventh) edition of the Tumor, Node, Metastasis Classification for Lung Cancer. *Journal of Thoracic Oncology*, **2** (12), 1067–1077.

Spiro, S.G., Gould, M.K. and Colice, G.L. (2007) American College of Chest Physicians. Initial evaluation of the patient with lung cancer: symptoms, signs, laboratory tests, and paraneoplastic syndromes: ACCP evidenced-based clinical practice guidelines (2nd edition). *Chest*, **132** (3 Suppl.), 149S–160S.

Further reading

BTS (2007) *Statement on Malignant Mesothelioma in the United Kingdom*, British Thoracic Society Standards of Care Committee. *Thorax*. **62**, ii1–ii19.

De Leyn, P., Lardinois, D., Van Schil, P.E., *et al.* (2007). ESTS guidelines for preoperative lymph node staging for non-small-cell lung cancer. *European Journal of Cardiothoracic Surgery*, **32** (1), 1–8.

Detterbeck, F.C., Boffa, D.J. and Tanoue, L.T. (2009) The new lung cancer staging system. *Chest*, **136**, 260–271.

NICE (2011) Guidance for lung cancer. Available at http://www.nice.org.uk/CG121NICEguideline. Accessed May 2010 in draft form.

Robinson, B.W. and Lake, R.A. (2005) Advances in malignant mesothelioma. *New England Journal of Medicine*, **353** (15), 1591–1603.

Silvestri, G.A., Gould, M.K., Margolis, M.L., *et al.* (2007) American College of Chest Physicians. Non-invasive staging of non-small-cell lung cancer: ACCP evidenced-based clinical practice guidelines (2nd edition). *Chest*, **132** (3 Suppl.), 178S–201S.

Spira, A. and Ettinger, D.S. (2004) Multidisciplinary management of lung cancer. *New England Journal of Medicine*, **350** (4), 379–392.

Wagner, J.C., Sleggs, C.A. and Marchand, P. (1960) Diffuse pleural mesothelioma and asbestos exposure in the North Western Cape Province. *British Journal of Industrial Medicine*, **17**, 260–271.

Chapter 3

Chemotherapy and Biological Agents

Fharat A. Raja and Siow Ming Lee

Key points

- There has been significant progress in the treatment of lung cancer in the last decade.
- Pemetrexed, gefitinib and erlotinib are the latest additions and have significantly improved survival as first-line, maintenance, and second-line treatments for advanced NSCLC.
- Histological determination and EGFR mutation testing are now routinely used to select patients for individualised treatment.

Introduction

The prognosis for patients with lung cancer has continued to remain poor over the last 25 years because most patients still present with advanced disease. Until a validated screening programme is available to detect early lung cancer in order to increase the resection rates and cures, the majority of these patients will be treated with chemotherapy with or without radiotherapy.

For the purpose of treatment, lung cancer is divided into non-small-cell lung cancer (NSCLC) and small-cell lung cancer (SCLC). NSCLC includes an aggregate of histologies (adenocarcinoma, squamous and large-cell) that historically have been approached in very similar ways with regard to diagnosis, staging and treatment. More recent data suggested that different histological types respond with varying degrees of success to cytotoxic and biological agents. We are now customising treatment plans on the basis of histology and genetic mutations.

Lung Cancer: A Multidisciplinary Approach, First Edition. Edited by Alison Leary.
© 2012 Blackwell Publishing Ltd. Published 2012 by Blackwell Publishing Ltd.

SCLC is staged and treated differently from NSCLC and its treatment options are considered separately.

Chemotherapy

Chemotherapy plays an important role in the treatment of lung cancer. In limited stage SCLC, chemotherapy is used with radiotherapy to attempt cure. For extensive stage, chemotherapy can induce significant disease response and remission although many patients will eventually relapse again. In NSCLC, chemotherapy further improves survival rate when used after curative resection.

For patients with advanced NSCLC, chemotherapy significantly improves 1-year survival, disease control and quality of life. NICE has recommended that chemotherapy should be offered to patients with stage III or IV NSCLC and good performance status (WHO 0, 1 or Karnofsky score of 80–100) and should be a combination of a single third-generation drug (docetaxel, gemcitabine, paclitaxel or vinorelbine) plus a platinum drug. Either carboplatin or cisplatin may be administered, taking into account their toxicities, efficacy and convenience. The range of toxicities is shown in Table 3.1.

A side effect not listed in Table 3.1 is *fatigue*, which every chemotherapy drug causes to a varying degree. This can be difficult to reverse and is independent of anaemia and other toxicities that may contribute to fatigue. Most chemotherapy drugs are used in combination, usually a platinum drug with another drug. Many clinicians favour carboplatin instead of cisplatin because it is less emetogenic and can be given as a short out-patient infusion without the requirement for pre- and post-treatment hydration. It must be emphasized that *neutropenic septicaemia* is the most dangerous life-threatening toxicity, which frequently occurs 7–14 days after treatment and must be treated immediately and aggressively with broad-spectrum antibiotics. Use of prophylactic antibiotics and G-CSF (granulocyte-colony stimulating factor) should also be considered with some of the myelosuppressive chemotherapy in order to prevent neutropenic deaths.

Who gets chemotherapy?

Many lung cancer patients are elderly and often have multiple co-morbidities and are therefore of poor performance status. For this reason, the number of patients in the UK who actually receive chemotherapy can be as low as 20% in SCLC patients (NHS IC 2009).

Many of these patients might benefit from single-agent chemotherapy with a third-generation drug as recommended by NICE (2011). It is hoped that with the introduction of multidisciplinary team meetings in many hospitals, more lung cancer patients will be offered treatment or be considered for clinical trials.

Table 3.1 Chemotherapy agents used in lung cancer.

Drug	Main side effects	Dose-limiting side effects	Additional comments
Cisplatin	Nausea and vomiting, myelosuppression, ototoxicity, neuropathy, electrolyte derangement	Nephrotoxicity	Requires long hydration time
Gemcitabine	Nausea and vomiting, flu-like symptoms, diarrhoea, oedema, rash	Myelosuppression	
Docetaxel	Oedema and fluid retention, nausea and vomiting, diarrhoea, alopecia, rash	Myelosuppression	Requires high-dose dexamethasone prior to, during and after infusion
Paclitaxel	Nausea and vomiting, myalgia, mucositis, peripheral neuropathy, hypersensitivity reaction, alopecia	Myelosuppression	Requires pre-treatment with dexamethasone
Vinorelbine	Nausea and vomiting, hair thinning	Myelosuppression	
Vincristine	Constipation, hair thinning	Neuropathy	Vesicant
Etoposide	Nausea and vomiting, mucositis, alopecia	Myelosuppression	
Pemetrexed	Nausea and vomiting, anaemia		Requires B_{12}, folic acid, dexamethasone treatment before and after infusion

Adjuvant treatment

The high rate of recurrence following resection for early NSCLC suggests that micrometastases already exist at the time of surgery. Data from a 1995 meta-analysis (NSCLC Collaborative Group 1995) suggested that trials using platinum-based chemotherapy might improve survival (hazard ratio (HR) 0.87, 95% confidence interval (CI) 0.74–1.02, $P = 0.008$). It was nearly a decade before randomised trials confirmed survival benefits in patients receiving adjuvant chemotherapy.

The International Adjuvant Lung Cancer Trial (Arriagada et al. 2004) randomised 1867 patients to cisplatin-based chemotherapy or to observation. All stages of NSCLC were represented, with 36.5% having pathological stage I disease, 24.2% stage II, and 39.3% stage III. The drug allocated with cisplatin was etoposide in 56.5% of patients, vinorelbine in 26.8%, vinblastine in 11.0%, and vindesine in 5.8%. Patients having chemotherapy had a statistically significant improvement in overall survival (44.5% vs 40.4% at 5 years, $P < 0.03$) and also disease-free survival (39.4% vs 34.3% at 5 years $P < 0.003$).

The ANITA (Adjuvant Navelbine International Trialist Association) trial also showed benefit in the adjuvant setting (Douillard et al. 2006). In this trial 840 patients were randomised to chemotherapy (cisplatin plus vinorelbine) or observation. Median survival was 65.7 months (95% CI 47.9-88.5) in the chemotherapy group and 43.7 (35.7-52.3) months in the observation group. Overall survival at 5 years with chemotherapy improved by 8.6%, which was maintained at 7 years (8.4%).

A third trial from Canada also demonstrated survival benefits (Winton et al. 2005). In this trial 482 patients were randomized to chemotherapy (vinorelbine and cisplatin) or observation. The 5-year survival was significantly greater in the chemotherapy arm compared with observation (69 vs 54%, $P = 0.03$). Severe toxicity was uncommon with less than 10% having common toxicity criteria grade 3 (ECOG 2007); there were two chemotherapy-related deaths.

Following the publication of these studies, adjuvant chemotherapy is generally offered to patients with good performance status. The statistical benefits reported are comparable to those seen in other solid malignancies including breast cancer. However, many lung cancer patients are older and have associated co-morbid problems unlike breast cancer patients, and may be less fit to receive adjuvant chemotherapy. Recommendation for chemotherapy should take into consideration how well the patients are likely to tolerate the chemotherapy. Patients should be encouraged to participate in clinical trials wherever possible so that the optimal chemotherapy regimen and/or the role of the new biological agents (e.g. erlotinib, bevacizumab) can be determined.

Neo-adjuvant treatment

Neo-adjuvant treatment refers to the use of chemotherapy prior to surgery with the aim of down-staging locally advanced cancer so that it is resectable and to reduce risk of metastases. However, there is a theoretical possibility that delaying definitive surgery with neo-adjuvant chemotherapy might prevent curative surgery due to disease progression.

Rosell et al. (1994) randomised 60 patients with IIIA NSCLC to surgery plus chemotherapy or surgery alone. Chemotherapy comprised three cycles of mitomycin, ifosfamide and cisplatin prior to surgery. Survival was significantly increased in the chemotherapy plus surgery arm at 26 months compared with 8 months in the surgery-alone arm ($P < 0.001$). Although these results were impressive, sample size was small and the surgery-alone arm did very poorly, with survival similar to that of metastatic disease. The same group published an updated analysis at 7 years (Rosell et al. 1999), which showed that the survival advantage persisted in the pre-op chemotherapy arm but the margin narrowed to a more modest 22 months versus 11 months ($P < 0.005$). In the pre-op chemotherapy arm, 32% of patients (8 out of 25) had evidence of tumour down-staging.

A second trial by Roth *et al.* published in the same year, randomized 60 patients with resectable stage IIIA NSCLC (Roth *et al.* 1994). Patients had six cycles of perioperative chemotherapy consisting of cyclophosphamide, cisplatin and etoposide. After three cycles of pre-op chemotherapy, 35% of patients had a major clinical response. Median survival of patients in the chemotherapy arm was 64 months compared with 11 months for patients who had surgery alone (*P* < 0.018). The authors also concluded that perioperative chemotherapy plus surgery was more effective than surgery alone.

Unfortunately, the two studies described were small and underpowered for any meaningful conclusion to be drawn. In an attempt to determine the role of neo-adjuvant chemotherapy, the MRC (LU 22 trial) conducted a large randomised trial (Gilligan *et al.* 2007). In this trial 519 patients were randomised to receive either surgery alone (*n* = 261) or chemotherapy followed by surgery (*n* = 258). Chemotherapy consisted of three cycles of platinum-based treatment at 3-weekly intervals. The authors concluded that no benefit was seen in overall survival for the neo-adjuvant arm (HR 1.02, 95% CI 0.80–1.31, *P* = 0.86). However, when the results of their trial were added to previous randomised trials for meta-analysis, they reported a 12% relative survival benefit with the addition of neo-adjuvant chemotherapy, which corresponded to a 5% absolute benefit at 5 years – very similar to that for patients receiving adjuvant chemotherapy. Trials comparing adjuvant versus neo-adjuvant chemotherapy are currently being planned to determine which schedule confers greater survival advantage. It is possible that the two approaches should be targeted to different populations. Gilligan *et al.* (2007) suggested using neo-adjuvant chemotherapy for those patients requiring down-staging preoperatively or for those patients in whom postoperative chemotherapy would be too difficult owing to co-morbidities. Until more trial data are available, the use of neo-adjuvant chemotherapy should be discussed within a multidisciplinary team (including oncologists and surgeons), on an individual-patient basis.

Chemotherapy for advanced NSCLC

Chemotherapy is the standard of care in locally advanced, unresectable NSCLC (i.e. stage IIIB and stage IV) for patients with good performance status. It can increase survival and improve symptoms associated with lung cancer. The first evidence suggesting a beneficial role of chemotherapy was a meta-analysis published in 1995 showing that cisplatin-based chemotherapy produced a small survival benefit (NSCLC Collaborative Group 1995). The Big Lung Trial was set up in the UK to confirm the survival benefits suggested by the meta-analysis (Spiro *et al.* 2004). It randomised 725 patients to receive either supportive care alone (*n* = 361) or supportive care plus cisplatin-based chemotherapy (*n* = 364). Patients allocated chemotherapy were found to have a statistically improved survival compared with no chemotherapy (8.0 months compared with 5.7 months; *P* = 0.0006). In addition, no significant differences were observed between the two groups in terms of predefined primary and secondary quality of life end points. It was found that any toxicity from chemotherapy was balanced by the improved palliation of pain and other symptoms.

The Eastern Cooperative Oncology Group (ECOG) conducted a randomised clinical trial to compare the efficacy of four commonly used third-generation regimens (Schiller *et al.* 2002). A total of 1207 patients with advanced non-small-cell lung cancer were randomly assigned to one of four regimens: cisplatin and paclitaxel, cisplatin and gemcitabine, cisplatin and docetaxel, or carboplatin and paclitaxel. The response rate for eligible patients was 19% with a median survival of 7.9 months. The response rate and survival did not differ significantly between patients assigned to any of the four regimens. The toxicity profiles did vary, but no particular regime stood out as being significantly better tolerated. In the UK, the London Lung Cancer group conducted a randomised trial comparing gemcitabine/carboplatin with MIC (mitomycin C, ifosfamide and cisplatin). This study demonstrated that gemcitabine/carboplatin was superior to MIC, increasing the median survival from 7.6 months to 10 months and 1-year survival from 30% to 40%, and was associated with less nausea, vomiting, constipation and alopecia, fewer admissions for administration, and better quality of life. This important study established gemcitabine/carboplatin as standard treatment of care in the UK and worldwide (Rudd *et al.* 2005).

Pemetrexed (Alimta) is a new multitargeted antifolate that inhibits thymidate synthase, dihydrofolate reductase and glycinamide ribinucleotide formyltransferase, and has an excellent safety profile and a convenient administration schedule (10-minute infusion). Pemetrexed is one of the standards of care for second-line treatment of NSCLC after showing comparable efficacy to docetaxel but with reduced toxicity (Hanna *et al.* 2004). Recently the combination of pemetrexed/cisplatin was found not to be inferior to gemcitabine/cisplatin overall as first-line treatment, but was better tolerated, with reduced toxicity profile including inducing significantly less neutropenia, anaemia, thrombocytopenia, febrile neutropenia and alopecia (Scagliotti *et al.* 2008). Interestingly, subgroup analysis showed that overall survival was statistically superior for cisplatin/pemetrexed versus cisplatin/gemcitabine in patients with adenocarcinoma (n = 847; 12.6 vs 10.9 months, respectively) and large-cell carcinoma histology (n = 153; 10.4 vs 6.7 months, respectively). In contrast, in patients with squamous cell histology, there was a significant improvement in survival with cisplatin/gemcitabine versus cisplatin/pemetrexed (n = 473; 10.8 vs 9.4 months, respectively). The survival of 12.6 months for adenocarcinoma histology is the highest reported for advanced NSCLC patients and with such a large number of patients included in the trial the results were accepted by the FDA, EMEA and NICE for approval of cisplatin/pemetrexed as first-line treatment of NSCLC with non-squamous histology.

Ciuleanu *et al.* examined the role of pemetrexed maintenance therapy in patients with stage IIB or IV NSCLC (Ciuleanu *et al.* 2008). All patients had been treated with a platinum doublet and had achieved at least stable disease. Patients were then randomised 2:1 to pemetrexed maintenance (500 mg/m^2 three-weekly) or to placebo. Patients on pemetrexed had a significantly greater progression-free survival than those on placebo (median progression-free survival 4.04 months versus 1.97 months, $P < 0.00001$). There was a trend towards improved overall survival with pemetrexed group having a median survival of 13 months versus 10 months in placebo ($P = 0.060$). However, analysis according to histological group showed greater progression-free survival and response rate in non-squamous NSCLC. This study resurrects the question of the role of maintenance therapy as previous studies did not demonstrate that more chemotherapy is better for patients with NSCLC.

Addition of targeted therapies to chemotherapy in NSCLC

With most cancer types there is always the possibility that adding more treatment may produce better response and survival. However, in NSCLC, triplet chemotherapy produced significantly increased toxicity and no benefits. Better understanding of the signalling pathways in lung cancer and the introduction of biological agents during the last decade has led to many biological trials combining these new drugs with standard chemotherapy. These trials focus mainly on the angiogenic and epidermal growth factor receptor signalling pathways.

Antiangiogenics

Angiogenesis is one of the hallmarks of cancer, and drugs to counteract this process have been shown to be effective in other malignancies, particularly in bowel cancer and renal cell cancer. For NSCLC, bevacizumab is now approved by the FDA and EMEA for the treatment of advanced NSCLC. This is based on the ECOG 4599 study, which demonstrated improved survival. This study randomised 878 patients with advanced non-squamous NSCLC to chemotherapy (carboplatin and paclitaxel) with bevacizumab or chemotherapy alone (Sandler et al. 2006). The median survival was 12.3 months in the bevacizumab arm and 10.3 months in the chemotherapy-alone group ($P = 0.003$). However, a European study combining bevacizumab with gemcitabine/cisplatin doublet (AVAiL) found only modest improved progression-free survival but no survival benefit (Manegold et al. 2007). In the UK, the London Lung Cancer Group examined the oral antiangiogenic drug thalidomide in combination with standard gemcitabine/carboplatin (Lee et al. 2009a). Here, 722 patients were randomised to receive placebo or thalidomide from the start of chemotherapy and then daily for up to 2 years. In this large trial, thalidomide in combination with chemotherapy did not improve survival, and was associated with an increased risk of a thrombotic event. The median overall survival was 8.9 months in placebo and 8.5 months with thalidomide. A similar finding was reported with sorafenib when combined with carboplatin and paclitaxel. These data add to a growing body of evidence that targeted antiangiogenic strategies in NSCLC may not be as effective as originally thought.

Anti-epidermal growth factor receptors: gefitinib, erlotinib and cetuximab

Epidermal growth factor receptors (EGFRs) play an important role in the growth and survival of many solid tumours, including NSCLC. EGFR is expressed in approximately 90% of NSCLC. EGFR can be antagonized by inhibition of intrinsic receptor tyrosine kinase activity by gefitinib or erlotinib (brand names Iressa and Tarceva, respectively) or with the monoclonal antibody cetuximab (Erbitux). Unlike single-agent clinical activity reported when used as second- and third-line treatment (Fukuoka *et al.* 2003), small-molecule EGFR inhibitors (gefitinib and erlotinib) when combined with standard doublet did not improve survival (Giaccone *et al.* 2004; Herbst *et al.* 2004, 2005; Gatzemeier *et al.* 2007). The reason for these negative studies is unclear but the results suggest an antagonism between chemotherapy and EGFR tyrosine kinase inhibitors when combined.

This is in contrast to the finding reported when erlotinib was used after standard chemotherapy. National Cancer Institute of Canada Clinical Trials Group Study BR.21 established erlotinib as a standard of care in patients with non-small-cell lung cancer after failure of first- or second-line chemotherapy (Shepherd *et al.* 2005). In this study involving 731 patients where 49% had received two prior chemotherapy regimens, and 93% had received platinum-based chemotherapy, erlotinib improved survival from 4.7 months to 6.7 months and also cancer-related symptoms compared with placebo. Erlotinib has been approved by the FDA and EMEA for second- and third-line treatment for NSCLC. This drug was approved by Scottish Medicines Consortium (SMC) for restricted use within NHS Scotland after failure of at least one prior chemotherapy regimen in patients who would otherwise be eligible for treatment with docetaxel chemotherapy. NICE has now given approval for erlotinib for the treatment of patients who would otherwise be eligible for treatment with second-line docetaxel chemotherapy.

NICE also recently approved gefitinib for first-line treatment of patients who have advanced or metastatic NSCLC and have tested positive for EGFR mutation. This is based on the Iressa Pan Asian Study (IPASS), demonstrating significant progression-free survival benefit for patients with EGFR mutation when treated with gefitinib compared with chemotherapy.

Cetuximab

Cetuximab (Erbitux) is approved by the EMEA and FDA for use in colorectal and head and neck cancers. Cetuximab in combination with cisplatin/vinorelbine was also recently demonstrated to improve survival for patients with advanced NSCLC (Pirker *et al.* 2008). Median survival reported for the combination was 11.3 months compared with 10.1 months for the chemotherapy-alone arm for the whole population. However, the median survival reported for the Asian subgroup was 17.6 months for the combination and 20.4 months for the chemotherapy alone. This is in contrast to the white population where the median survival was 10.5 months and 9.1 months for the combination and chemotherapy, respectively. There are several problems with this study, including the fact that cisplatin/vinorelbine is perceived as an inferior regimen compared to the taxane regimens; high neutropenic and infection rates (grade III/IV neutropenia 50% and febrile neutropenia 22% in the combination arm); and a selected population after screening 1861 NSCLC patients with only 1125 patients randomised into the study. At the present moment, it is unlikely that Erbitux will be adopted widely by lung cancer clinicians to treat advanced NSCLC until a confirmatory trial involving a newer chemotherapy regimen is able to show survival benefits.

New agents

Another promising class of novel agents being investigated in NSCLC is that of drugs targeting against insulin-like growth factor receptor type 1 (IGF-1R). A recently reported phase II trial of CP-751871, a monoclonal antibody against IGF-1R, with carboplatin and paclitaxel found the combination was well tolerated, with 46% responding to treatment (Karp *et al.* 2007). The drug is now undergoing a phase III trial and results are awaited with interest.

Chemotherapy for small-cell lung cancer

Small-cell lung cancer, 15–20% of all lung cancer, has been recognised as a unique subtype of lung cancer since the 1960s. Without treatment, the median survival is extremely poor, ranging from 2 to 4 months. Its clinical and biological characteristics exhibit very aggressive behaviour and are also frequently associated with paraneoplastic syndromes. However, it is exquisitely sensitive to chemotherapy and radiotherapy. For this reason, SCLC patients with poor performance status should be offered chemotherapy. There has been little progress in the treatment of small-cell lung cancer in the last few decades and the standard chemotherapy remains a platinum-based chemotherapy (such as cisplatin or carboplatin) in combination with etoposide.

The generally accepted staging for small-cell lung cancer divides all cases into limited stage and extensive stage (Table 3.2).

The chemosensitivity of SCLC was initially shown in a study using alkylating agents in these patients in the 1960s (Green *et al.* 1969). Striking responses were seen in patients treated with cyclophosphamide alone. With combination chemotherapy, response rates average 60–80%. Unfortunately, most patients eventually relapse again.

Since the 1980s, the standard of care for SCLC has been the combination of cisplatin and etoposide (Evans *et al.* 1985). Carboplatin can be substituted for cisplatin in elderly patients, in extensive disease, or in those with renal

Table 3.2 Staging of small-cell lung cancer – a system still in common clinical use for decision making in treatment of SCLC although this may change with the advent of TNM staging for SCLC (Shepherd *et al.* 2007).

| Limited stage | Confined to one hemithorax. Ipsilateral pleural effusion. Nodal involvement | 40% |
| Extensive stage | Metastatic lesions in contralateral lung. Distant metastases (brain, bone, liver, adrenals etc.) | 60% |

impairment, without loss of efficacy (Okamoto 2005). Numerous trials have been performed to test the newer agents – epirubicin, gemcitabine, the taxanes, ifosfamide and vinorelbine – but none has been found to improve survival. More intensive regimens with three or more drugs produced more toxicity without improving survival. Oral etoposide monotherapy, used frequently in the past for patients with poor performance status, is not as effective as combination and should therefore be avoided.

Attempts to improve survival including increasing treatment cycles beyond the standard 4–6 cycles, maintenance chemotherapy treatment, alternating chemotherapy schedules, dose intensification including high-dose chemotherapy with peripheral stem cell rescue, have all to date failed to improve survival. Other approaches include combining thalidomide, an antiangiogenic agent, with standard chemotherapy, which was also recently reported by the London Lung Cancer Group not to improve survival.

Limited stage small-cell lung cancer

Combination chemotherapy together with mediastinal radiotherapy and prophylactic cranial irradiation (PCI) remains the cornerstone of treatment for limited stage small-cell lung. This multimodality approach cures approximately 15–25% of limited stage SCLC patients. Perry *et al.* (1987) randomised patients between chemotherapy alone, chemotherapy plus delayed radiotherapy, or chemotherapy plus concurrent radiotherapy. All their patients also received prophylactic cranial irradiation. Statistically significant benefit was seen in local control, failure-free survival and overall survival in the two radiotherapy arms. Prophylactic whole-brain radiotherapy should be offered to all patients who have achieved an excellent partial response or complete remission. A meta-analysis of seven PCI trials involving 987 patients demonstrated a 5.4% overall survival benefit at 3 years. In addition, there was a reduction in incidence of brain metastases from 59% to 33% (Auperin 1999).

Extensive stage small-cell lung cancer

Combination chemotherapy is the mainstay of treatment for patients with extensive stage SCLC. Carboplatin/etoposide combination is frequently used to treat these poor-prognosis patients, improving their median survival from

4-6 weeks to 9-10 months. Other combinations have also been extensively investigated during the last decade. The combination of irinotecan plus cisplatin was initially reported to have achieved better survival by the Japanese group (Noda *et al*. 2002) (median survival 12.8 months vs 9.4 months, $P = 0.002$) but this study was not confirmed in two randomised trials performed in the United States (Hanna *et al*. 2006; Natale *et al*. 2008). In a UK-based trial, 241 patients with extensive stage and poor-prognosis limited stage small-cell lung cancer were randomised to receive gemcitabine and carboplatin or etoposide and cisplatin (Lee *et al*. 2009b). Results showed similar survival, but patients receiving cisplatin/etoposide reported more alopecia, nausea and cognitive impairment. Gemcitabine and carboplatin produced more myelosuppression but this was not associated with increased sepsis, hospital admissions or fatalities.

Extensive stage SCLC patients should also be treated with PCI after achieving significant disease response with chemotherapy. This was based on a European Organisation for Research and Treatment of Cancer study demonstrating a significant reduction in the risk of developing brain metastases in the patients receiving PCI (Slotman *et al*. 2007). The 1-year survival rates were 27% with PCI compared with 13% in the control group ($P = 0.003$; HR 0.68, 95% CI 0.52-0.88).

Second-line treatment in small-cell lung cancer

Unfortunately, the majority of SCLC patients will relapse. Treatment of these patients is difficult and prognosis remains very poor. Recommendation varies in different cancer centres in the UK. Many oncologists generally assess patients' performance status, duration of response and extent of response to initial chemotherapy before recommending a management plan. In patients achieving significant response, having good performance status, and more than 3 months after completing primary chemotherapy, some clinicians may re-challenge the patients with the same chemotherapy. Others may consider second-line CAV chemotherapy (cyclophosphamide, doxorubicin and vincristine). Response rates reported vary from 8% to 28% in studies (Shepherd *et al*. 1987; Sculier *et al*. 1990). Topotecan was recently found to be effective as well as second line treatment (O'Brien *et al*. 2006; Eckardt 2007).

Mesothelioma

Malignant pleural mesothelioma is a locally invasive cancer that is almost always fatal. In the UK, 2000 deaths were recorded in 2005. Mesothelioma is linked to asbestos exposure in approximately 90% of all cases (Vogelzang *et al*. 2003; NICE 2008). The incidence of mesothelioma has been estimated to continue to rise until 2015, following which the numbers will begin to fall, reflecting a time lag from the highest use of asbestos in the 1970s.

Most mesothelioma patients present with advanced disease, so curative surgical resection is not an option. Patients often have multiple symptoms and require active management of chest pain, dyspnoea and excess pleural fluid.

A variety of combination and single-agent regimens have been used to treat mesothelioma over the years but no single regimen has been considered the gold standard until now. In January 2008, NICE recommended pemetrexed as a treatment option for malignant mesothelioma. This was based on the results of the EMPHACIS trial ('Evaluation of Mesothelioma in a Phase 3 trial of Pemetrexed with Cisplatin') (NICE 2008). A total of 448 chemonaive patients were randomised to pemetrexed and cisplatin ($n = 226$) or cisplatin alone ($n = 222$). Patients were eligible if their Karnofsky performance status was greater than or equal to 70 (WHO performance status 0-1) and had a minimum life expectancy of 12 weeks. In the early stages of the trial there were three treatment-related deaths in the first 43 patients in the pemetrexed/cisplatin arm. In addition, other incidences of severe toxicity were noted. After 117 patients had been enrolled into the trial, folic acid and vitamin B_{12} supplementation were added to both treatment arms. This resulted in a significant reduction in toxicity in the pemetrexed/cisplatin arm. The primary end point of the trial was survival and median survival in the combination arm was significantly prolonged: 12.1 months versus 9.3 months in the control arm ($P = 0.02$). The tumour response rate was also significantly greater in the pemetrexed/cisplatin arm: 5.7 months versus 3.9 months ($P = 0.001$). This important trial has established pemetrexed and cisplatin as the standard treatment for good performance status patients in the UK.

A second trial compared cisplatin alone with raltitrexed plus cisplatin (Van Meerbeeck et al. 2005). Raltitrexed is an antimetabolite with pure and specific thymidine synthase inhibitor effect. It had demonstrated activity in mesothelioma in the phase II setting. A total of 250 patients were randomised to single-agent cisplatin or raltitrexed in combination with cisplatin. All patients had no prior chemotherapy and were of performance status 0-2. The response rate in the cisplatin/raltitrexed arm was 23.6% compared with 13.6% in the cisplatin-alone arm ($P = 0.056$). Median overall survival was 11.4 months and 8.8 months ($P = 0.048$) for combination versus single agent treatment. There was no difference in quality of life assessments in both arms. In conclusion, the effect seen with the combination of raltitrexed and cisplatin is similar to that seen with pemetrexed and cisplatin and therefore confirms that doublet chemotherapy is superior to single-agent treatment in malignant mesothelioma.

A third trial, mainly based in the UK, randomised 409 patients with malignant mesothelioma to active symptom control (ASC) ($n = 136$) or chemotherapy plus ASC (Muers et al. 2005). ASC involved regular follow-up in specialist clinics and use of steroids, analgesics, appetite stimulants, bronchodilators or palliative radiotherapy as required. The chemotherapy arms consisted of MVP (mitomycin, vinblastine and cisplatin) ($n = 137$) or vinorelbine alone ($n = 136$). because of slow accrual following licensing of pemetrexed, the trial design was changed and the two chemotherapy groups were combined. Overall survival was not significantly prolonged in the chemotherapy arm (8.5 months) versus the ASC-alone arm (7.6 months) (HR 0.89, 95% CI 0.72-1.10; $P = 0.29$). When the two chemotherapy arms were considered separately, patients in the vinorelbine arm had a longer overall survival than those in the ASC group (HR 0.80, 95% CI 0.63–1.02; $P = 0.08$). No benefit was seen when ASC alone group was compared with the MVP group (HR 0.99, 95% CI 0.78–1.27; $P = 0.95$). Comparison of the two chemotherapy groups directly gave a hazard ratio of 0.77 (95% CI 0.61–0.99; $P = 0.04$), suggesting a benefit of vinorelbine compared with MVP.

The trials described above are the largest randomised trials in malignant mesothelioma. In light of the results, pemetrexed has been licensed for use in patients of good performance status with malignant mesothelioma. Future progress may lie in using novel agents either alone or in combination with chemotherapy.

Summary

There has been significant progress in the treatment of lung cancer in the last decade. Pemetrexed, gefitinib and erlotinib are the latest additions and have significantly improved survival as first-line and second-line treatments for advanced NSCLC. We are now approaching an era of histological determination and EGFR mutation testing to select patients for the optimum treatment.

References

Arriagada, R., Bergman, B., Dunant, A., *et al.* (2004) International Adjuvant Lung Cancer Trial Collaborative Group. Cisplatin-based adjuvant chemotherapy in patients with completely resected non-small-cell lung cancer. *New England Journal of Medicine*, **350** (4), 351–360.

Auperin, A., Arriagada, R., Pignon, J.P., *et al.* (1999) Prophylactic cranial irradiation for patients with small-cell lung cancer in complete remission. Prophylactic Cranial Irradiation Overview Collaborative Group. *New England Journal of Medicine*, **341** (7), 476–484.

Ciuleanu, T.E., Brodowicz, T., Belani, C.P., *et al.* (2008) Maintenance pemetrexed plus best supportive care (BSC) versus placebo plus BSC: a phase 3 study. *Journal of Clinical Oncology*, **26** (Suppl.), abstract 8011.

Douillard, J.Y., Rosell, R., De Lena, M., *et al.* (2006) Adjuvant vinorelbine plus cisplatin versus observation in patients with completely resected stage IB–IIIA non-small-cell lung cancer (Adjuvant Navelbine International Trialist Association [ANITA]): a randomised controlled trial. *Lancet Oncology*, **7** (9), 719–727.

Eckardt, J.R., von Pawel, J., Pujol, J.L., *et al.* (2007) Phase III study of oral compared with intravenous topotecan as second-line therapy in small-cell lung cancer. *Journal of Clinical Oncology*, **25**, 2086–2092.

ECOG (2007) *Common Toxicity Criteria* (short form). Eastern Cooperative Oncology Group. Available at: http://ecog.dfci.harvard.edu/general/ctc.pdf. Accessed July 2011.

Evans, W., Shepherd, F., Field, R., *et al.* (1985) VP-16 and cisplatin as first-line therapy for small-cell lung cancer. *Journal of Clinical Oncology*, **3**, 1471–1477.

Fukuoka, M., Yano, S., Giaccone, G., *et al.* (2003) Multi-institutional randomized phase II trial of gefitinib for previously treated patients with advanced non-small-cell lung cancer (The IDEAL 1 Trial) *Journal of Clinical Oncology,* **21** (12), 2237–2246.

Gatzemeier, U., Pluzanska, A., Szczesna, A., *et al.* (2007) Phase III study of erlotinib in combination with cisplatin and gemcitabine in advanced non-small-cell lung cancer: the Tarceva Lung Cancer Investigation Trial. *Journal of Clinical Oncology,* **25** (12), 1545–1552.

Giaccone, G., Herbst, R.S., Manegold, C., *et al.* (2004) Gefitinib in combination with gemcitabine and cisplatin in advanced non-small-cell lung cancer: a phase III trial – INTACT 1. *Journal of Clinical Oncology,* **22** (5), 777–784.

Gilligan, D., Nicolson, M., Smith, I., *et al.* (2007) Preoperative chemotherapy in patients with resectable non-small-cell lung cancer: results of the MRC LU22/NVALT/EORTC 08012 multicentre randomised trial and update of systematic review. *Lancet,* **369**, 1929–1937.

Green, R.A., Humphrey, E., Close, H., *et al.* (1969) Alkylating agents in bronchogenic carcinoma. *American Journal of Medicine,* **46**, 516–525.

Hanna, N., Shepherd, F.A., Fossella, F.V., *et al.* (2004) Randomized phase III trial of pemetrexed versus docetaxel in patients with non-small-cell lung cancer previously treated with chemotherapy. *Journal of Clinical Oncology,* **22** (9), 1589–1597.

Hanna, N., Bunn, P.A. Jr, Langer, C., *et al.* (2006) Randomized phase III trial comparing irinotecan/cisplatin with etoposide/cisplatin in patients with previously untreated extensive-stage disease small-cell lung cancer. *Journal of Clinical Oncology,* **24** (13), 2038–2043.

Herbst, R.S., Giaccone, G., Schiller, J.H., *et al.* (2004) Gefitinib in combination with paclitaxel and carboplatin in advanced non-small-cell lung cancer: a phase III trial – INTACT 2. *Journal of Clinical Oncology,* **22** (5): 785–794.

Herbst, R.S., Prager, D., Hermann, R., *et al.* (2005) TRIBUTE: A phase 3 trial of erlotinib combined with carboplatin and paclitaxel chemotherapy in advanced non-small-cell lung cancer. *Journal of Clinical Oncology,* **23**, 5892–5899.

Karp, D.D., Paz-Ares, L.G., Blakely, L.J., *et al.* (2007) Efficacy of the anti-insulin like growth factor I receptor (IGF-IR) antibody CP-751,871 in combination with paclitaxel and carboplatin as first-line treatment for advanced non-small-cell lung cancer (NSCLC). *Proceedings of the American Society for Clinical Oncology,* **25**, 386s. Abstract 7506.

Lee, S.M., Rudd, R., Woll, P.J., *et al.* (2009a) Randomized double-blind placebo-controlled trial of thalidomide in combination with gemcitabine and carboplatin in advanced non-small-cell lung cancer. *Journal of Clinical Oncology,* **27** (31), 5248–5254.

Lee, S.M., James, L.E., Qian, W., *et al.* (2009b) Comparison of gemcitabine and carboplatin versus cisplatin and etoposide for patients with poor-prognosis small-cell lung cancer. *Thorax,* **64** (1), 75–80.

Manegold, C., von Pawel, J., Zatloukal, P., *et al.* (2007) Randomised, double-blind multicentre phase 3 study of bevacizumab in combination with cisplatin and gemcitabine in chemotherapy-naïve patients with advanced or recurrent non-squamous non-small-cell lung cancer (NSCLC) [ASCO Annual Meeting Proceedings Part I]. *Journal of Clinical Oncology,* **25** (18 June 20 Suppl.).

Muers, M.F., Stephens, R.J., Fisher, P., *et al.* (2005) Active symptom control with or without chemotherapy in the treatment of patients with malignant pleural mesothelioma (MS01): a multicentre randomised trial. *Lancet,* **371** (9625), 1685–1694.

Natale, R., Lara, P.N., Chansky, J., *et al.* (2008) S0124: A randomised phase III trial comparing irinotecan/cisplatin (IP) with etoposide/cisplatin (EP) in patients with previously untreated extensive stage small-cell lung cancer. *Journal of Clinical Oncology*, **26** (May 20 Suppl.), abstract 7512.

NHS Information Centre National Lung Cancer Audit (2009). Available at http://www.ic.nhs.uk/webfiles/Services/NCASP/audits%20and%20 reports/7089_Lung_Cancer_V5.pdf. Accessed 30 June 2011.

NICE (2008) *Pemetrexed Disodium for the Treatment of Malignant Pleural Mesothelioma*. NICE technology appraisal guidance 135. National Institute for Health and Clinical Excellence, London.

NICE (2011) Guidance for Lung Cancer CG 121 NICE Guidelines accessed October 2011.

Noda, K., Nishiwaki, Y., Kawahara, M., *et al.* (2002) Irinotecan plus cisplatin compared with etoposide plus cisplatin for extensive small-cell lung cancer. *New England Journal of Medicine*, **346** (2), 85–91.

Non-small-Cell Lung Cancer Collaborative Group (1995) Chemotherapy in non-small-cell lung cancer: a meta-analysis using updated data on individual patients from 52 randomised clinical trials. *British Medical Journal*, **311**, 899–909.

O'Brien, M.E.R., Ciuleanu, T.E., Tsekov, H., *et al.* (2006) Phase III trial comparing supportive care alone with supportive care with oral topotecan in patients with relapsed small-cell lung cancer. *Journal of Clinical Oncology*, **24**, 5441–5447.

Okamoto, H., Watanabe, K., Kunikane, H., *et al.* (2005) Randomised phase 3 trial of carboplatin (C) plus etoposide (E) vs split doses of cisplatin (P) plus etoposide (E) in elderly or poor risk patient with extensive disease small-cell lung cancer. *Journal of Clinical Oncology*, **23**, 623s.

Perry, M.C., Eaton, W.L., Propert, K.J., *et al.* (1987) Chemotherapy with or without radiation therapy in limited small-cell lung carcinoma of the lung. *New England Journal of Medicine*, **316** (15), 912–918.

Pirker, R,. Szczesna, A., von Pawel, J., *et al.* (2008) FLEX: A randomized, multicenter, phase III study of cetuximab in combination with cisplatin/vinorelbine (CV) versus CV alone in the first-line treatment of patients with advanced non-small-cell lung cancer (NSCLC). *Journal of Clinical Oncology*, **26** (May 20 Suppl.), abstract 3.

Rosell, R., Gómez-Codina, J., Camps, C., *et al.* (1994) A randomized trial comparing preoperative chemotherapy plus surgery with surgery alone in patients with non-small-cell lung cancer. *New England Journal of Medicine*, **330** (3), 153–158.

Rosell, R., Gomez-Codina, J., Camps, C., *et al.* (1999) Preresectional chemotherapy in stage IIIA non-small-cell lung cancer: a 7-year assessment of a randomized controlled trial. *Lung Cancer*, **26**, 7–14.

Roth, J.A., Fossella, F., Komaki, R., *et al.* (1994) A randomized trial comparing perioperative chemotherapy and surgery with surgery alone in resectable stage IIIA non-small-cell lung cancer. *Journal of the National Cancer Institute*, **86**, 673–680.

Rudd, R.M., Gower, N.H., Spiro, S.G., *et al.* (2005) Gemcitabine plus carboplatin versus mitomycin, ifosfamide, and cisplatin in patients with stage IIIB or IV non-small-cell lung cancer: a phase III randomized study of the London Lung Cancer Group. *Journal of Clinical Oncology*, **23** (1), 142–153.

Sandler, A., Gray, R., Perry, M.C., *et al.* (2006). Paclitaxel-carboplatin alone or with bevacizumab for non-small-cell lung cancer. *New England Journal of Medicine*, **355**, 2542–2550.

Scagliotti, G., Purvish, P., von Pawel, J., *et al.* (2008) Phase 3 study of pemetrexed plus cisplatin versus gemcitabine plus cisplatin in chemonaive patients with locally advanced or metastatic non-small-cell lung cancer (NSCLC). *Journal of Clinical Oncology*, **26** (21), 3543–3551.

Schiller, J.H., Harrington, D., Belani, C.P., *et al.* (2002) Comparison of four chemotherapy regimens for advanced non-small-cell lung cancer. *New England Journal of Medicine*, **346** (2), 92–98.

Sculier, J.P., Klastersky, J., Libert, P., *et al.* (1990) A phase 2 study evaluating CAV potentiated or not by amphotericin B entrapped into sonicated liposomes, as salvage therapy for small-cell lung cancer. *Lung Cancer*, **6**, 110–118.

Shepherd, F.A., Evans, W.K., Maccormick, R., *et al.* (1987) Cyclophosphamide, doxorubicin and vincristine in etoposide and cisplatin-resistant small-cell lung cancer. *Cancer Treatment Reports*, **71**, 941–944.

Shepherd, F.A., Rodrigues Pereira, J., Ciuleanu, T., *et al.* (2005) National Cancer Institute of Canada Clinical Trials Group. Erlotinib in previously treated non-small-cell lung cancer. *New England Journal of Medicine*, **353** (2), 123–132.

Shepherd, F., Crowley, J., Van Houtte, P., *et al.* (2007) The International Association for the Study of Lung Cancer Lung Cancer Staging Project: Proposals Regarding the Clinical Staging of Small-Cell Lung Cancer in the Forthcoming (Seventh) Edition of the Tumor, Node, Metastasis Classification for Lung Cancer. *Journal of Thoracic Oncology*, **2** (12), 1067–1077.

Slotman, B., Faivre-Finn, C., Kramer, G., *et al.* (2007) Prophylactic cranial irradiation in extensive small-cell lung cancer. *New England Journal of Medicine*, **357**, 664–672.

Spiro, S.G., Rudd, R.M., Souhami, R.L., *et al.* (2004), Chemotherapy versus supportive care in advanced non-small-cell lung cancer: improved survival without detriment to quality of life. *Thorax*, **59**, 828–836.

Van Meerbeeck, J.P., Gaafar, R., Manegold, C., *et al.* (2005) European Organisation for Research and Treatment of Cancer Lung Cancer Group; National Cancer Institute of Canada. Randomized phase III study of cisplatin with or without raltitrexed in patients with malignant pleural mesothelioma: an intergroup study of the European Organisation for Research and Treatment of Cancer Lung Cancer Group and the National Cancer Institute of Canada. *Journal of Clinical Oncology*, **23** (28), 6881–6889.

Vogelzang, N.J., Rusthoven, J.J., Symanowski, J., *et al.* (2003) Phase III study of pemetrexed in combination with cisplatin versus cisplatin alone in patients with malignant pleural meothelioma. *Journal of Clinical Oncology*, **21**, 2636–2644.

Winton, T., Livingston, R., Johnson, D., *et al.* (2005) National Cancer Institute of Canada Clinical Trials Group; National Cancer Institute of the United States Intergroup JBR.10 Trial Investigators. Vinorelbine plus cisplatin vs. observation in resected non-small-cell lung cancer. *New England Journal of Medicine*, **352** (25), 2589–2597.

Chapter 4
Lung Radiotherapy

Nita Patel and Dawn Carnell

Key points

- Radiotherapy is an important modality of treatment in lung cancer patients.
- Radiotherapy is planned carefully to minimise side-effects and morbidity.
- Radiotherapy is an important tool in providing symptom control.

Introduction

It is important that the management of lung cancer is multidisciplinary. Surgery, chemotherapy and radiotherapy, and supportive care all play an integral part in the management of lung cancer.

Radiotherapy is used in the management of both non-small-cell and small-cell lung cancer. It can be used in an attempt to cure the primary lung cancer (known as radical radiotherapy), and can also be used to palliate symptoms (palliative radiotherapy).

This chapter will focus on the principles of radiotherapy and the role it plays in the management of lung cancer.

Principles of radiotherapy

History of radiotherapy

X-rays were discovered by Roentgen in 1895. This discovery sparked a great deal of interest and they were soon put to use in industry and medicine. In 1902 it was reported that dramatic shrinkage of bulky Hodgkin disease was

Lung Cancer: A Multidisciplinary Approach, First Edition. Edited by Alison Leary.
© 2012 Blackwell Publishing Ltd. Published 2012 by Blackwell Publishing Ltd.

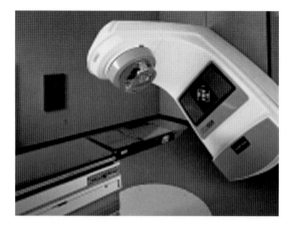

Fig. 4.1 Clinac linear accelerator. (Image courtesy of Varian Medical Systems, Inc. All rights reserved.)

achieved using these newly discovered X-rays. However, the limitations of the crude X-ray tubes available in those early years resulted in early local systemic relapse. Over the years, many technological advances have been made in the delivery of ionising radiation. These, along with a better understanding of how radiation works and radiobiological principles, have established the crucial role that radiotherapy plays in the management of a wide range of malignancies.

In 1951, the first treatment using high-energy radiotherapy was given in London, Canada using a cobalt machine (Johns *et al.* 1951). Cobalt-60 machines use a radionuclide as the source of ionising radiation. These machines were simple and reliable to use, and enabled the clinician to deliver high-energy radiation in a reliable and safe manner. However, there are many disadvantages to cobalt machines, the most important being the widening of the radiation field edge. This means that a larger area of the patient is treated than is desirable, making the treatment less accurate. Another important disadvantage of this form of radiation delivery is that the source of radiation is a decaying radioactive source that needs to be changed approximately every 5 years. This means that the treatment delivery time increases as the source gets older. Henry Kaplan and his colleagues developed the linear accelerator in the late 1950s in Stanford. The linear accelerator, or linac as it is commonly known, can produce a large, penetrating and accurate beam (Fig. 4.1). This permits higher doses of radiation to be given to more precisely delineated target volumes, and enables smaller volumes of normal tissue to be irradiated.

In recent years, the advent of three-dimensional computed tomography (3D-CT)-based planning has further enabled the clinician to delineate the target volume more accurately. CT planning also allows more accurate definition of critical structures, and dose calculation. 3D planning, as well as the use of shaped alloy blocks, allows improved levels of conformation. Multileaf collimators consist of small symmetrical leaves made of tungsten alloy that present in large numbers on a linear accelerator. The leaves are driven out automatically and independently of each other to shape the volume to be treated. This allows shaping of the high-dose target volume as closely as possible, allowing sparing of normal tissues. They are also used in IMRT (intensity modulated radiotherapy). IMRT can produce complex treatment volumes that closely conform to the target volume. This can allow dose escalation to the tumour and reduction of normal tissue doses.

How does radiotherapy work?

Radiotherapy is the use of ionising radiation to produce cell kill. Radiation can be considered as packets of energy in the form of photons (X-rays, gamma rays) or particles (protons, neutrons, electrons). Radiation deposits energy in tissue and produces ionisation events, and this can either be directly ionising radiation (charged particles) or indirectly ionising radiation (X-rays and gamma rays). The radiation dose is the term that describes the quantity of energy deposited per unit mass of tissue. The standardised international unit of absorbed dose is the *gray* (Gy). This is defined as the absorbed dose of radiation per unit mass in a medium, and 1 Gy is equal to 1 joule per kilogram (1 J/kg).

Radiation kills cells by producing secondary charged particles and free radicals in the cell nucleus, which in turn produce a variety of DNA damage. DNA is damaged by two processes, direct and indirect damage, with indirect damage predominating. High-energy X-rays collide with orbital electrons of biological molecules, causing ejection of electrons. These can directly damage DNA or can produce hydroxyl radicals (OH^-) from water molecules in tissues, which in turn cause DNA damage. Radiation causes several types of DNA damage. A dose of 1–2 Gy can cause more than 1000 base damages, about 1000 single-strand breaks, and about 40 double-strand breaks. Studies have shown that double-strand DNA breaks are the lethal event. Cells may die immediately, but most commonly proceed to mitosis and undergo mitotic death. Clonogenic cells have infinite proliferative capacity, and it is the loss of these cells that leads to tumour eradication. Therefore, the higher the dose of radiation, the higher the cell kill from double-strand DNA damage, and the higher the loss of clonogenic cells. This then leads to a greater chance of eradicating tumour. However, owing to normal tissue tolerance, it is not possible to give unlimited doses of radiation to kill tumour cells as that will cause irreversible damage to normal cells, leading to death.

Similarly, it is not possible to give single large doses of radiation, as this will also irreversibly damage normal tissue. Instead, the radiotherapy dose is given in smaller doses at each administration, i.e. the total dose is spilt into smaller doses per session. This is known as fractionation. An example of a fractionated dose schedule in lung cancer is 64 Gy in 32 fractions (64 Gy/32#), which equates to 2 Gy per fraction. When the number of fractions is increased or the dose per fraction is decreased, then the total dose required to produce the same amount of cell kill is increased. However, this is more desirable, as use of greater fractionation and lower doses per fraction allows recovery of normal tissues from sublethal DNA damage and produces a better therapeutic index. In other words, it maximises tumour cell kill and minimises damage of normal cells.

Methods of delivery of radiation treatment

As mentioned earlier, ionising radiation can be in the form of directly ionising radiation comprising charged particles, or indirectly ionising radiation such as X-rays. In the treatment of malignant disease there are two main methods of delivery of ionising radiation to the tumour cells, and these can use both direct and indirect ionising sources.

Brachytherapy is the use of radioactive sources implanted directly into, or adjacent to, the tumour. The combining term *brachy* is derived from the Greek meaning 'short' (distance). Several different radioactive sources can be used. Some examples include caesium-137, iodine-125 and iridium-192. Radioactive sources can emit X-rays, gamma rays or beta rays depending on the source. These in turn can cause indirect or direct ionisation.

The other mode of delivery is called **external beam radiotherapy**. This is treatment with beams of ionising radiation produced from a source external to the patient. There are three forms of external beam radiotherapy; Electron beam, orthovoltage, and megavoltage therapy. Orthovoltage machines produce low-energy X-ray beams, and these are used to treat superficial tumours because the dose of radiation is deposited within a few centimetres of the skin. They are a form of indirect ionising radiation. Electron beam therapy can also be used to treat superficial tumours; this a form of direct ionising radiation. It is delivered using a linear accelerator. Megavoltage X-rays are defined as > 1MV, and are used to treat deeper-seated tumours. This is because the maximum dose is deposited below the skin surface, and this also allows skin sparing. The majority of linear accelerators are 6MV in energy, but 10MV machines are also commonplace. Machines of 4MV and 15MV are also available but are less commonly used.

Medical linear accelerators

A linear accelerator is a large machine (Fig. 4.2) that can produce both electron and X-ray beams. The components of the machine include the stand, gantry, treatment head and treatment couch. The stand is fixed to the floor, and is connected to the power supply. The gantry moves around the patient through 360°, and the treatment head is attached to the end of it.

High-energy X-rays are produced by using electromagnetic fields to propel charged particles to great energies. Electrons are emitted from a heated gun filament, and electromagnetic waves (microwaves) are then used to accelerate the electrons and increase their energy. The microwave power is transmitted by hollow tubes called waveguides. The beam of electrons is steered through an angle of approximately 90° to focus the beam. They then hit a heavy-metal

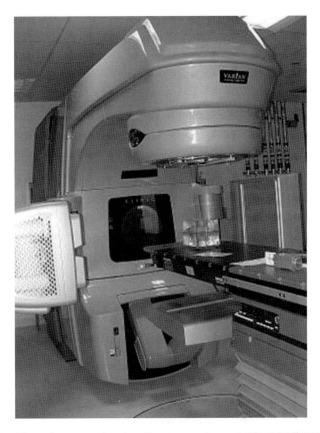

Fig. 4.2 Clinac linear accelerator. (Image courtesy of UCLH NHS FT.)

X-ray target. The X-ray beam that is produced is collimated through a primary collimator. The intensity of the beam is made more uniform by use of a flattening filter. The next component of the treatment head is the secondary collimator, which has four jaws and also houses the multileaf collimators. These four jaws can move independently from one another and can produce asymmetric beams.

The majority of modern linear accelerators have a dual purpose, as stated earlier, and can produce X-rays and electron beams. Electron beams are produced by removing the X-ray target and replacing it with a scattering foil. The final step in producing an electron beam is attachment of an applicator to the treatment head. This minimises scattering of the electrons.

Radiotherapy planning

The aim of radiotherapy is to achieve a high dose of radiation to the target volume and minimise the dose to normal tissues. To achieve this, radiotherapy treatment is planned very carefully and the planning process is an important part in ensuring that this is achieved. There are several steps in the planning process, and these will now be described in more detail.

Preparation

Patients are generally discussed in a multidisciplinary team (MDT), and the treatment plan is decided using clinical information, imaging and histo-pathology results. This allows accurate staging of the tumour, and encourages discussion about the individual patient to formulate a management plan that is suitable for that patient. This is crucial, as a patient with a lung cancer that is resectable on the grounds that it is an early stage tumour may not be resectable because of their poor lung function or performance status. In cases such as these, the MDT may decide that radiotherapy is the best course of action. The clinician then needs to decide the treatment intent, i.e. radical or palliative radiotherapy. Palliative radiotherapy is given to provide symptomatic relief. The planning and delivery of radiotherapy is usually a simple technique, and the doses that are used are smaller and are given over a shorter period of time. In palliative radiotherapy, since the aim is to provide symptomatic relief, the acute side effects of radiotherapy are less acceptable but the long-term side effects may not be relevant. This is because the prognosis may be months, so the patient is unlikely to live long enough to develop any long-term toxicity. In radical radiotherapy the radiation dose is designed to cure the tumour. These are more complex treatment plans with more sophisticated radiotherapy techniques. Radical radiotherapy is usually planned using 3D-CT treatment planning systems. As the aim of treatment is to obtain long-term cure, the risk of long-term side effects is not acceptable, but the risk of acute side effects might be.

Once the decision to treat with radiotherapy has been made, and the treatment intent decided, the patient needs to be seen in an out-patient setting. The decision to treat will be finalised at that stage, and informed consent obtained.

Patient positioning

The position of the patient is important, as changes in position during radiotherapy and between each fraction can result in over- or underdosage. The position should be comfortable for the patient, should be reproducible, and should allow localisation of the tumour without the radiotherapy beams entering or exiting through unrelated structures. An example of this is the arms, which should be positioned away from the trunk in chest radiotherapy to ensure that the radiotherapy beams do not unnecessarily irradiate the arms. Patients are usually positioned supine on the treatment couch, as this is the most comfortable position. The patient is then immobilised using a variety of techniques. This is crucial, because without immobilisation patients will change their position, making the treatment less accurate. For radiotherapy to the brain, patients are immobilised using a thermoplastic shell. This is a specially designed plastic mould that is made pliable by immersion in hot water. It can then be moulded around the patient's face to produce an individualised mask for immobilisation. In lung radiotherapy, patients also have moulds made of their trunk for immobilisation. Additional methods of immobilisation include a head rest, knee rest and ankle stocks.

Tumour localisation

The localisation of the target volume must be done in the same conditions as the subsequent treatments. There are three methods of localising the target volume. The target volume can be defined clinically, which is called mark on-set. This is mainly used for skin cancers because the tumour is easily visible. In lung cancer, radiotherapy can be used to treat the port-site (site of biopsy) in patients with mesothelioma because the target volume includes the scar and the biopsy tract. A simulator is a machine similar to the linear accelerator which can reproduce treatment conditions. There are the treatment couch, gantry and lasers, but it has a diagnostic quality X-ray machine that allows a simple method of localising the area that needs to be treated. It is used for palliative treatments as it provides a quick and easy way identify the target volume. For radical radiotherapy, patients have a CT scan to delineate the target volume. The planning CT scan differs from a diagnostic CT scan. The couch is flat-topped, and the patient lies in the treatment position using immobilisation techniques and laser lights. The CT scanner is also connected to a treatment planning machine, allowing direct transfer of the CT images. The use of CT images provides anatomical information that then allows delineation of the target volume more accurately and also avoidance of critical structures. Once the patient is positioned in the simulator or CT scanner, reference tattoos are placed on the skin to aid tumour localisation. A tattoo is made on the skin over the nearest bony landmark in the centre of the target volume, and additional lateral tattoos are placed to prevent lateral rotation. In palliative treatments, patients may not require as many tattoos. In brain radiotherapy, the tattoos are placed on the mask to avoid marking the patient's skin. These skin tattoos act as reference points, and the laser positioning lights are used to align the patient using these reference points.

Tumour volume definition

The International Commission for Radiological Units (ICRU 1993, 1999) recommends international definitions of tumour, target and normal organ volumes for comparison of clinical results.

The gross tumour volume (GTV) is defined as the macroscopic extent of the tumour that is palpable, visible or detectable using imaging. A margin around the GTV is given to account for any potential microscopic disease around the tumour, and this may include any potential lymph node(s) that may harbour microscopic deposits. The volume that includes the GTV and margin to account for microscopic spread is called the clinical target volume (CTV). The planning target volume (PTV) is the final volume and is the volume that the treatment is planned on. This volume has a margin to account for uncertainties and variations in treatment. The volume to be treated will vary during treatment because of organ motion, and this is particularly marked in lung radiotherapy as respiration will make the volume to be treated move during the treatment. A margin must be added to account for this. There will also be variations in the positioning of the patient on a day-to-day basis, and also in the alignment of the beams, so a margin also needs to be added to account for these. These margins are added to the CTV to form the PTV, and the PTV should get 95% of the prescribed dose of radiation.

In simulator planning, it can be difficult to define these volumes. However, it should be easy to define the GTV using diagnostic imaging and these margins should be added to produce the PTV. A further margin needs to be added, as the target volume that is defined in the simulator is the field. The field is the area that receives 50% of the dose, and a margin of 15 mm on the PTV usually suffices to obtain this. In CT planning, these volumes are defined, and any organs at risk are also outlined. These volumes are then sent to planning physics and a treatment plan is produced using a treatment planning machine.

Arrangement of radiotherapy beams

The next step in planning a patient's radiotherapy is to decide on the number and direction of the radiotherapy beams. This differs depending on the site to be treated and also the treatment intent. Palliative radiotherapy is usually delivered with a single treatment field or an opposed field, as this allows simplicity in planning, delivery of radiotherapy and dose calculation. A simple one- or two-field radiotherapy plan does not need to be sent to physics for planning, and the fields are defined in the simulator (Fig. 4.3). Palliative radiotherapy to the lung is usually treated with an anterior and posterior field, although for high-dose palliative radiotherapy multiple fields can be used. Parallel opposed fields are also used in whole-brain radiotherapy. In parallel opposed fields, the dose is prescribed to the mid-plane dose. A single field is usually prescribed to a depth, or alternatively as an applied dose. Single fields are commonly used in treating the spine for either bone pain or spinal cord compression. Multiple fields are used for radical radiotherapy, but can also be used for high-dose palliative lung radiotherapy. Usually three fields are used, but more complex field arrangements might be required to ensure adequate coverage of the PTV. The central axis of these beams passes through one point, which is known as the isocentre. The isocentre is placed in the centre of the PTV, and the beam arrangements are chosen to avoid dose entering or exiting critical structures. However, it can be impossible to avoid critical structures completely, and in these cases the aim is to ensure as little dose to these sensitive structures as possible. Each organ at risk has a tolerance, and the aim of planning is to ensure that the organs receive less than the tolerance dose. Radical lung radiotherapy plans that require multiple beams are sent to planning physics to obtain an optimal plan. The treatment is prescribed to

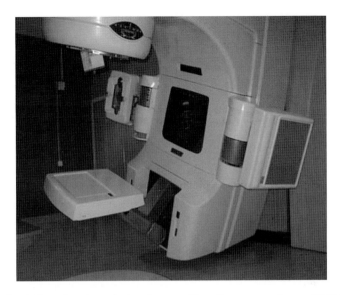

Fig. 4.3 Eclipse treatment planning machine. (Image courtesy of UCLH NHS FT.)

100%, and the plan should have a dose range between 95% and 107%. Dose volume histograms (DVHs) are also produced as part of the final plan. These give parameters of the volume of the PTV that receives different dose levels. In addition to giving the dose range of the PTV, DVHs of the organs at risk are also given.

Implementation and verification

Once the radiotherapy has been planned, it is important to ensure that all the parameters of treatment such as field size, wedges and shielding are checked and that the dose prescription is correct. Once the patient starts their treatment it is important to make sure that there are no major variations in set-up and this is done by using electronic portal imaging. These are radiographs that are taken while the patient is on the treatment couch in the treatment position. These are then compared with the images on which patient has been planned. In the majority of cases, these will be taken after the first three fractions of radiotherapy, and then weekly thereafter. If there are any problems with set-up, this will need to be accounted for.

The use of radiotherapy in non-small-cell lung cancer

Radiotherapy has a major role to play in the management of non-small-cell lung cancer. Radical radiotherapy can be used as a treatment modality in stage I–III NSCLC. Palliative radiotherapy can also be used in these stages, as well as in stage IV disease. Palliative radiotherapy will be described in more detail in another section. Postoperative radiotherapy has previously been out of favour, but it is now coming back into use. There have also been trials looking at the use of neo-adjuvant chemotherapy, concomitant chemoradiation, and also the use of continuous hyperfractionated accelerated radiotherapy (CHART) These will now be described in more detail.

Radical radiotherapy in NSCLC

The median age at presentation for lung cancer in the UK is over 70 years. Many of these patients will have smoking-related co-morbidities such as emphysema and cardiovascular disease. This means that a number of patients may be medically inoperable. Surgery should be considered in all patients with either stage I or stage II NSCLC, but because of these factors it may not always be feasible. In this setting, these patients should be considered for radical radiotherapy. In this setting, these patients should be considered for radical radiotherapy. Patients undergoing radical radiotherapy require adequate lung function, but the level of FEV_1, FVC and transfer factor is not as defined or limiting as it is for surgical patients. There are no strict rules about what level of lung function is necessary, but the location and size of the tumour are important in dictating the level of lung function that you would accept. If the tumour is peripheral, you may accept a lower level of FEV_1 and transfer factor. This is because the volume of lung that will be in the treated field will be less than if the tumour were more central. Treating smaller tumours will also mean that less of the lung will be in the treated field, and you may accept a lower lung function. However, patients with a $FEV_1 < 1L$ and transfer factor $< 50\%$ should be treated with caution.

Patients with stage III NSCLC can be considered for surgery if they have a small primary lymph node or resectable mediastinal lymph nodes. However, the majority of patients with stage III NSCLC are treated with radical radiotherapy if they are suitable. Suitable patients would include those with:

- A good performance status
- Adequate lung function
- No significant co-morbidities and minimal weight loss

The volume of disease should also be such that it can be treated to a high enough dose without a high risk of radiation pneumonitis. Radiation pneumonitis will be described in a later section.

Standard UK practice would involve treating the disease in either a single phase or two phases, without prophylactic radiotherapy to the mediastinal lymph nodes. The doses that are commonly used are 55 Gy in 20 fractions over 4 weeks in a single phase, or 64 Gy in 32 fractions over 6½ weeks using one or two phases. Patients undergoing conventional radiotherapy do not have any treatment over the weekend, and will generally have five fractions per week.

Radical radiotherapy with chemotherapy

Combined modality therapy is standard for stage III NSCLC. Patients usually receive sequential chemotherapy. i.e. 3–4 cycles of platinum-based chemotherapy prior to radiotherapy. There have been several trials investigating sequential chemotherapy with radiotherapy, and there is some evidence to suggest that there is a survival advantage (Dillman *et al.* 1990; Pritchard and Anthony 1996). However, the size of this benefit is unclear. Concurrent chemotherapy with radiotherapy has also been shown to be effective in several trials, and a recent meta-analysis of nine published and unpublished trials has shown that there is a 4% survival advantage at 2 years in favour of concurrent platinum-based chemotherapy compared with radiotherapy alone (Aupérin *et al.* 2006). There is an increase in toxicity with concurrent chemoradiation, particularly oesophagitis. Several trials have compared concurrent versus sequential chemotherapy, and there is some evidence to suggest that chemotherapy given concurrently with radiotherapy may be more effective than sequential chemotherapy (Furuse *et al.* 1999; Curran *et al.* 2003). Currently sequential chemotherapy is commonly used to manage stage III NSCLC out of the trial setting. This allows down-staging of the tumour and enables the disease to be encompassed in a radical radiotherapy volume.

Continuous hyperfractionated accelerated radiotherapy

In continuous hyperfractionated accelerated radiotherapy (CHART), the treatment time and dose per fraction are decreased and the number of fractions is increased. Hyperfractionation is the use of doses per fraction less than the conventional 1.8–2 Gy. This means that the total number of fractions is increased, and at least two fractions of radiotherapy are administered per day, at least six hours apart. The advantage of this is that the incidence of late-responding normal tissue damage is less with a lower dose per fraction, and it allows dose escalation. Acceleration is defined as shortening of the overall treatment time, or increasing the total dose per week above the conventional 10 Gy. It follows from this that patients undergoing CHART are given a dose higher than 10 Gy per week in doses per fraction that are less than 1.8 Gy with more than one fraction administered per day at least six hours apart. A randomised trial compared CHART with conventional radiotherapy (Saunders *et al.* 1999); 563 patients were randomised to either conventional radiotherapy using 60 Gy in 30 fractions, or to CHART. The doses that were given in CHART were 54 Gy in 36 fractions, 1.5 Gy per fraction over 12 days with no treatment gap over the weekend. Patients were given three fractions per day. This trial showed that there was a significant benefit in the 5-year overall survival in patients undergoing CHART. The 5-year overall survival (OS) was 29% in the CHART arm compared with 20% in the conventional arm, and this difference was more marked in those patients with a squamous cell carcinoma. The OS benefit at 5 years in these patients was 14%. Oesophagitis occurred earlier and was more significant in the CHART group, but there were no long-term concerns. Therefore, CHART is recommended in the treatment of NSCLC where possible. However, it is logistically difficult to administer owing to the continuous nature of the treatment and the necessity for administering three treatments a day, which means that patients are required to stay in hospital for the duration of their treatment. All these factors make CHART a difficult treatment modality to deliver, and it is available only in selected centres in the UK.

Postoperative radiotherapy

Adjuvant postoperative radiotherapy (PORT) can theoretically be used in an attempt to eradicate microscopic residual tumour deposits, but unfortunately the results from trials attempting to answer this question have been variable. A large meta-analysis published in 1998 pooled data from nine published and unpublished trials that randomised postoperative radiotherapy versus surgery alone (PORT Meta-analysis Trialists Group 1998). This trial showed that the routine use of PORT had a detrimental effect, and the 2-year overall survival was reduced by 7% in the PORT group, from 55% to 48%. This survival disadvantage could possibly be accounted for by the late effects on the heart and lung in long-term survivors in the PORT arm. A subgroup analysis showed that the decreased survival was mainly in the N0 and N1 patients. It also showed that patients with N2 or N3 disease had improved local control but no improvement in survival. This trial has been criticised, however, as the trials included were old and used older radiotherapy techniques and dose schedules that are not relevant to the modern-day practice. Current recommendations would be to consider PORT in patients who have gross residual disease or positive or close resection margins, or in those patients with mediastinal lymph nodes.

The doses that can be used include 55 Gy in 20 fractions or 64 Gy in 32 fractions for gross residual disease, or alternatively 50 Gy in 25 fractions or 60 Gy in 30 fractions for microscopic residual disease.

The use of radiotherapy in small-cell lung cancer

Small-cell lung cancer is a chemosensitive disease and, in almost all cases, the initial management is with chemotherapy. In patients with extensive stage SCLC, there is no role for thoracic irradiation except to palliate symptoms. However, recent evidence suggests that patients with extensive stage SCLC who have a good response to chemotherapy will benefit from prophylactic cranial irradiation (PCI). This will be described in more detail below. Limited stage SCLC is treated with chemotherapy. If there is a good response to chemotherapy, then the patient will proceed to both thoracic irradiation and PCI. The evidence for this will now be described in more detail.

Thoracic irradiation in SCLC

As mentioned earlier, there is not enough evidence to support the use of thoracic irradiation (TI) in extensive stage SCLC. However, it is routinely used to treat patients with limited stage SCLC. It is important to assess a patient's performance status, as it may not be appropriate to treat a patient with a poor performance status with radiotherapy.

Trials have shown that TI can improve 3-year survival by 5.4% (Pignon *et al.* 1992; Warde and Payne 1992), but the timing of radiotherapy with chemotherapy can be controversial. There is evidence to suggest that early concurrent radiotherapy delivered after the first or second cycle of chemotherapy confers a survival benefit (Murray *et al.* 1993; De Ruysscher *et al.* 2006). However, this is a more toxic regimen, and the survival advantage is only maintained if the optimal dose intensities of both the chemotherapy and radiotherapy are achieved. For these reasons, the timing of radiotherapy varies between centres.

The optimal dose of radiotherapy has not been established, but there is evidence to suggest that twice-daily treatment over 15 days provides a survival advantage (Turrisi *et al.* 1999). The dose that is given in this regime is 45 Gy in 30 fractions, with twice-daily fractions given at least 6 hours apart. The limitation of this dose regimen is that it is more toxic than once-daily fractionation regimes and it also causes an extra burden on the treatment machines. In the UK, the most common fractionation regimes use 15 fractions. The dose can vary, and doses of 40 Gy or 45 Gy in 15 fractions are widely used.

Prophylactic cranial irradiation

Approximately 50% of patients with SCLC will develop brain metastases within 2 years. In patients who have limited stage SCLC and in whom the primary thoracic disease is controlled, the brain becomes one of the main sites of relapse. The theory behind this is that the brain becomes a sanctuary site because of the inability of cytotoxic drugs to cross the blood–brain barrier. This led to several trials looking at the role of prophylactic cranial irradiation (PCI) in limited stage SCLC. In these trials, a small decrease in the incidence of brain metastases was demonstrated, but it was not until a seminal meta-analysis was published in 1999 that PCI came into widespread use (Aupérin *et al.* 1999). This meta-analysis demonstrated that there was as 5.4% 3-year survival benefit in giving patients with limited stage SCLC prophylactic cranial irradiation. The doses that were used varied, as did the fractionation. The most commonly used dose and fractionation schedule is 25–30 Gy in 10 fractions. PCI is delivered after both chemotherapy and thoracic irradiation, and there should be a gap of at least 2 weeks between completion of thoracic irradiation and PCI.

Despite the knowledge that brain metastases are common in SCLC and the conclusive role of PCI in limited stage SCLC, it was not until 2007 that the technique found a role in extensive stage SCLC. In one study patients with extensive stage SCLC who had a good response to chemotherapy received PCI, and it was found that the 1-year survival rate improved by 13.7% (Slotman 2009). The doses that were used were 20 Gy in 5 fractions and 30 Gy in 10 fractions. Based on this evidence, 20 Gy in 5 fractions is now given to all patients with extensive stage SCLC who have a good response to chemotherapy.

Palliative radiotherapy

Palliative radiotherapy is used in both NSCLC and SCLC. It has a more limited role in SCLC as the mainstay of treatment is chemotherapy, even in palliation. However, it can be used in patients who have intractable local symptoms despite chemotherapy, or in patients who have progressed during chemotherapy. In NSCLC, palliative lung radiotherapy is used more commonly, and can be used in patients who have local symptoms such as haemoptysis, chest pain and cough. It is not so good in palliating dyspnoea or lethargy. Palliative radiotherapy is also used to manage spinal cord compression, brain metastases and bone pain in both NSCLC and SCLC.

Palliative lung radiotherapy

The use of palliative radiotherapy to the lung is important, as it provides good symptomatic relief. Traditionally higher dose and fractionation regimes were used. A dosage of 30 Gy in 10 fractions was a commonly used dose schedule. The problem with this was that patients with advanced lung cancer have a poor prognosis, so bringing them up to the radiotherapy department for 2 weeks is not ideal. In addition, radiotherapy was not thought to confer a survival benefit, and was only given to palliate symptoms. Three trials in the 1990s provided a great deal of information on palliative radiotherapy to the lung. A regimen of 30 Gy in 10 fractions was compared with 17 Gy in 2 fractions given over 1 week (MRC Lung Cancer Working Party 1991). This showed that there was no difference in survival or palliation of symptoms. Another trial compared the 17 Gy in 2 fractions schedule with 10 Gy in one fraction in patients with a poor performance status (MRC Lung Cancer Working Party 1992). This also did not show any difference in survival or palliation. However, 10 Gy in one fraction can be quite toxic if the area to be treated is large. In cases such as these, 20 Gy in 5 fractions is a good alternative. In patients with a good performance status, a trial comparing 17 Gy in 2 fractions with 39 Gy in 13 fractions showed that there was a 2-month survival advantage with the high-dose palliative regime (MRC Lung Cancer Working Party 1996). It is important to plan high-dose palliative radiotherapy using 3D conformal techniques, as otherwise the dose to critical structures including the spinal cord and normal lung will be exceeded beyond tolerance.

Therefore, patients who have a poor performance status should receive 10 Gy in one fraction or 20 Gy in 5 fractions if the field is large. Patients with a good performance status should receive 39 Gy in 13 fractions where possible.

Palliative brachytherapy

Intraluminal brachytherapy can be used to treat patients who have previously received external beam radiotherapy to the lung. The radioactive source that is used is high-dose iridium-192. A bronchoscopy is performed to determine the proximal and distal limits of the tumour and this is recorded on radiographs with a measuring grid. The tumour length is then defined using a guide wire and a margin of 1 cm is added on either end. The guide wire is removed and the iridium source is then introduced. Brachytherapy to the bronchus is usually delivered in one treatment.

Radiotherapy for brain metastases

If a patient with either NSCLC or SCLC develops brain metastases, then the initial management will be to give whole-brain radiotherapy. This is to prevent further neurological deterioration and to wean the patient off steroids. The patient will then proceed to chemotherapy or lung radiotherapy depending on what is the next best step in their management. The dose used is 20 Gy in 5 fractions, and this is given over 1 week. If a patient who has previously received whole-brain radiotherapy either as PCI or for symptomatic brain metastases requires further radiotherapy to the brain, it might be possible to deliver this. This will depend on the time interval between the initial treatment and the new presentation; not only does this give a guide to the natural history of the disease, but a longer time interval also allows recovery of normal brain tissue. The patient should also be re-staged, as it may not be appropriate to re-treat the brain if the patient has widespread metastatic disease. The dose that is used on re-treatment depends on the initial dose. If the patient received a 10-fraction regimen as part of PCI then it would be safe to give 20 Gy in 5 fractions. However, if the patient received 20 Gy in 5 fractions as part of their initial treatment it would be safer to give the repeat treatment over 2 weeks using a 10-fraction dose schedule.

Radiotherapy for spinal cord compression and bony metastases

Spinal cord compression is an oncological emergency. Patients should be started on 16 mg dexamethasone once a day if there is clinical suspicion of spinal cord compression, and they should also be given medication for gastroprotection. The patient should then have MRI of the whole spine to confirm the diagnosis. Once this has been performed, the patient should be given palliative radiotherapy to the relevant vertebral levels to prevent further neurological deterioration. The most common dose used to treat spinal cord compression is 20 Gy in 5 fractions, but 8 or 10 Gy in one fraction can also be used. Palliative radiotherapy is also be used to treat sites of bony pain from bony metastases. A dosage of 20 Gy in 5 fractions used to be a common dose and fractionation schedule. However, trials have shown that 8 Gy in one fraction provides similar palliation and is now the most commonly used dose to treat bony metastases (Price *et al*. 1986; Steenland *et al*. 1999). Patients who do not respond to this dose can be re-treated using 20 Gy in 5 fractions, with good effect.

Management of patients during radiotherapy

Patients undergoing radiotherapy for lung cancer can have a wide range of symptoms and side effects, depending on the site that is irradiated and the dose that they are receiving.

All patients having radical lung radiotherapy over either 4 or 6½ weeks should be reviewed regularly. Usually they are reviewed weekly by a specialist radiotherapy nurse who has experience in managing patients undergoing radiotherapy. Patients are reviewed by a doctor in the first and last week of radiotherapy, and also once in the middle of their treatment. The toxicity of treatment is documented and graded, and the treatment card is reviewed to ensure that there are no discrepancies between the dose the patient has received and the expected toxicity. Patients usually do not develop any side effects until after the second week of radiotherapy, and the effects of treatment are cumulative, i.e. the severity of the side effects gets progressively worse as the treatment progresses. The side effects may get more severe for a couple of weeks after radiotherapy has been completed, and patients are warned and reassured about this. Patients receiving palliative radiotherapy are usually not reviewed as frequently, mainly because the treatment is given over a much shorter period, usually one or two weeks or even in one fraction. This means that they usually do not develop any toxicity during their radiotherapy and they may not develop any significant side effects at all. If they do have any effects, they usually manifest a week or so after completion of radiotherapy. Again, the patient should be warned of this. If a patient is having palliative radiotherapy over one or two weeks, they are usually reviewed on the last day of treatment. Patients are seen daily by the treatment radiographers, and if they or the patient are concerned about any new symptom, then they can be reviewed ad hoc.

Side effects of radiotherapy

The side effects of radiotherapy can be classified as acute or late. Acute toxicity is defined as any side effect that manifests itself within 90 days of starting radiotherapy. The acute effects are usually self-limiting and resolve within 6 weeks of completion of treatment. Late toxicity is any side effect that develops after 90 days. The late effects are usually permanent, and can develop many years after completion of radiotherapy. One of the aims of radiotherapy planning is to minimise the dose to the organs at risk, and thereby reduce the risk of long-term toxicity. All organs at risk have a tolerance dose, and these doses have been defined using animal models (Emami *et al*. 1991). The tolerance dose is the dose at which the risk of developing any given toxicity, e.g. myelopathy, is 5% at 5 years. It follows from this that doses lower than the tolerance dose, or doses that are within tolerance, may still produce the unwanted toxicity. When obtaining consent for radiotherapy the common side effects and the rarer but more serious effects need to be explained to the patient.

Acute side effects and how to manage them

The acute side effects from radiotherapy can either be general to radiotherapy or specific to the site that is being treated. General effects that occur in almost all patients undergoing radiotherapy are lethargy, skin erythema and hair loss in the treated area. The cause of lethargy is not fully understood but may have a multifactorial origin. Management of lethargy would include trying to exclude an organic cause such as anaemia.

Skin erythema can cause itchy, dry skin. The patient should be advised on skin care, which should include advising the patient not to use perfumed soaps and to keep out of the sun. Aqueous cream should be applied to the irradiated area at least twice a day. Depending on the area to be irradiated, the patient should also be warned of hair loss in the treated area. This is particularly relevant for patients receiving whole-brain radiotherapy. Hair loss is usually reversible, but patients who receive higher doses should be warned that the hair loss may be permanent.

Acute side effects from lung radiotherapy

The acute effects from radiotherapy to the lung will vary depending on the part of the lung being treated, the volume that is treated, and the total dose received. The potential acute side effects include:

- Dry cough
- Oesophagitis
- Hoarse voice
- Indigestion
- Nausea and vomiting
- Poor appetite

All these side effects should be treated with the appropriate medication. Dry cough can be managed with simple cough linctus, and if this does not control symptoms then either codeine linctus or even oral morphine solution may used. Oesophagitis is managed with sucralfate and analgesia. Indigestion and nausea may be controlled using antiemetics or a proton pump inhibitor. A hoarse voice is self-limiting, and the patient should be reassured. A poor appetite may respond to antiemetics or a proton pump inhibitor if nausea and/or indigestion are the cause. If the patient is losing a significant amount of weight, they may require high-energy supplemental feeding. If this becomes a significant problem, they should be referred to a dietician.

Acute side effects from whole-brain radiotherapy

The side effects of skin erythema and hair loss have already been mentioned above. They are the two main acute side effects from whole-brain radiotherapy. Some patients may also suffer from self-limiting somnolence 4–6 weeks after completion of radiotherapy.

Acute side effects from palliative radiotherapy to the spine or bone

Patients having a single fraction or even five fractions of radiotherapy for bony metastases rarely get any significant acute side effects other than lethargy and skin erythema. However, patients having treatment to the spine for spinal cord compression may suffer from additional side effects, depending on the vertebral levels that are being treated. These may include:

- Oesophagitis (cervical spine)
- Dry cough (thoracic spine)
- Indigestion (lower thoracic spine)
- Nausea and vomiting (lower thoracic and/or lumbar spine)
- Diarrhoea (lumbar and/or sacral spine)

These side effects should be managed with the appropriate medication.

Long-term toxicity and its management

The long-term toxicity from palliative radiotherapy to the spine for bone pain is unlikely to become relevant, as patients are not likely to live long enough to develop any long-term toxicity. The incidence of myelopathy caused by radiotherapy to the spinal cord is rare, but when it does occur there is unfortunately no specific treatment. The potential long-term effects from whole-brain radiotherapy were addressed in a meta-analysis investigating the potential benefit of prophylactic cranial irradiation in SCLC (Aupérin et al. 1999). However, only two out of the seven trials performed neuropsychological evaluation. There was no conclusive evidence that patients who received whole-brain radiotherapy developed any significant long-term memory deficit.

The most significant long-term side effect from lung radiotherapy is radiation pneumonitis. This usually occurs 8–12 weeks after completion of treatment. The risk of developing pneumonitis increases as the dose that the normal lung receives increases. A trial published by Graham et al. in 1999 demonstrated the incidence of pneumonitis with the V20 (Graham et al. 1999). This is illustrated in Table 4.1. The V20 is the volume of normal lung that receives 20 Gy, and in practical terms the aim is to keep this below 30%. However, there is still a risk of developing radiation pneumonitis if the V20 is over 22%. The severity of pneumonitis is graded as: Grade 1 – mild dyspnoea; Grade 2 – requiring steroids; Grade 3 – requiring O_2; Grade 4 – requiring ventilation.

Table 4.1 The risk of developing pneumonitis in proportion to V20, the volume of lung that receives 20 Gy (Graham *et al*. 1999).

V20	Grade 2 pneumonitis
<22%	0%
22–31%	7%
32–40%	13%
>40%	36%

Reprinted from *International Journal of Radiation Oncology, Biology, Physics*, Sep. 1; **45** (2), Graham M.V. *et al*. Clinical dose-volume histogram analysis for pneumonitis after 3D treatment for non-small-cell lung cancer (NSCLC), pp. 323–329 (1999) with permission from Elsevier.

Patients who develop radiation pneumonitis should be managed with 60 mg prednisolone and oxygen.

Other long-term side effects from lung radiotherapy include lung fibrosis, which may be asymptomatic but can cause increased breathlessness. There is no specific management other than symptomatic management, i.e. increased use of inhalers or oxygen as necessary.

Oesophageal stricture is a rare side effect, and may necessitate surgery to relieve the stricture.

New techniques under evaluation

Respiratory gating is a technique that is currently under investigation for use in radical radiotherapy planning and treatment. It images the tumour throughout the breathing cycle to allow an estimation of the tumour movement with breathing. This can inform about the margins that are used for radiotherapy; also, if the patient can cope with respiratory coaching to make their breathing controlled and reproducible, treatment can be given at a specific phase in the respiratory cycle. This can mean a reduction in the amount of healthy lung tissue that receives significant radiation dose and therefore a reduction in side effects may be possible.

Stereotactic lung radiotherapy is another radical treatment technique undergoing clinical evaluation. In contrast to conventional radiotherapy many beams of radiation are directed at the cancer. This treatment tends to be limited in its scope because it is only really suitable for relatively small peripheral lung cancers, as treatment needs to be targeted using the help of implanted fiducial markers. The dose is usually given in much larger fraction sizes over just a few days, making it much easier for the patient. The long-term results of this treatment are encouraging, however. With careful respiratory gating it may be possible to utilise this technique in more patients without the need for fiducial markers, which can be risky in this group of patients with often limited respiratory reserve.

Summary

Radiotherapy is a common treatment modality in the management of lung cancer and is used in the radical or the palliative setting. It can be used to palliate symptoms from either local or metastatic disease. However, it is important to manage the side effects of radiotherapy so as to maintain quality of life and manage morbidity.

References

Aupérin, A., Arriagada, R., Pignon, J.P., *et al.* (1999) Prophylactic cranial irradiation for patients with small-cell lung cancer in complete remission. Prophylactic Cranial Irradiation Overview Collaborative Group. *New England Journal of Medicine*, **341** (7), 476-484.

Aupérin, A., Le Pechoux, C., Pignon, J.P., *et al.* on behalf of the Meta-Analysis of Cisplatin/carboplatin based Concomitant Chemotherapy in non-small-cell Lung Cancer (MAC3-LC) Group. (2006) Concomitant radio-chemotherapy based on platin compounds in patients with locally advanced non-small-cell lung cancer (NSCLC): a meta-analysis of individual data from 1764 patients. *Annals of Oncology*, **17**, 473–483.

Curran, W.J., Scott, C.B., Langer, C.J., *et al.* (2003) Long-term benefit is observed in a phase III comparison of sequential vs concurrent chemoradiation for patients with unresected stage III nsclc: RTOG 9410 (abstract 2499). *Proceedings of the American Society for Clinical Oncology*, **22**, 621.

De Ruysscher, D., Pijls-Johannesma, M., Vansteenkiste, J., Kester, A., Rutten, I., Lambin, P. (2006) Systematic review and meta-analysis of randomised, controlled trials of the timing of chest radiotherapy in patients with limited-stage, small-cell lung cancer. *Annals of Oncology*, **17**, 543–552.

Dillman, R.O., Seagren, S.L., Propert, K.J., *et al.* (1990) A randomized trial of induction chemotherapy plus high-dose radiation versus radiation alone in stage III non-small-cell lung cancer. *New England Journal of Medicine*, **323**, 940-945.

Emami, B., Lyman, J., Brown A., *et al.* (1991) Tolerance of Normal Tissue to therapeutic irradiation. *International Journal of Radiation Oncology, Biology, Physics*, **21** (1), 109-122.

Furuse, K., Fukuoka, M., Kawahara, M., *et al.* (1999) Phase III study of concurrent versus sequential thoracic radiotherapy in combination with mitomycin, vindesine, and cisplatin in unresectable stage III non-small-cell lung cancer. *Journal of Clinical Oncology*, **17**, 2692-2699.

Graham, M.V., Purdy, J.A., Emami, B., *et al.* (1999) Clinical dose-volume histogram analysis for pneumonitis after 3D treatment for non-small-cell lung cancer (NSCLC). *International Journal of Radiation Oncology, Biology, Physics*, **45** (2), 323-239.

International Commission for Radiological Units (1993; 1999) *ICRU 50: Prescribing, Recording, and Reporting Photon Beam Therapy*. International Commission for Radiological Units; ICRU 62: *Prescribing, Recording and Reporting Photon Beam Therapy* (Supplement to ICRU Report 50). International Commission for Radiological Units, Bethesda, MD.

Johns, H.E., Bates L.M., Epp E.R., *et al.* (1951) 1,000-curie cobalt 60 units for radiation therapy. *Nature*, **168** (4285), 1035-1036.

Medical Research Council Lung Cancer Working Party (1991) Inoperable non-small-cell lung cancer (NSCLC). A Medical Research Council (MRC) randomised trial of palliative radiotherapy with two fractions or ten fractions. *British Journal of Cancer*, **63**, 265-270.

Medical Research Council Lung Cancer Working Party (1992) A Medical Research Council (MRC) randomised trial of palliative radiotherapy with two fractions or a single fraction in patients with inoperable non-small-cell lung cancer (NSCLC) and poor performance status. *British Journal of Cancer*, **65** (6), 934-941.

Medical Research Council Lung Cancer Working Party (1996) Randomized trial of palliative two-fraction versus more intensive 13-fraction radiotherapy for patients with inoperable non-small-cell lung cancer and good performance status. *Clinical Oncology (R Coll Radiol)*, **8**(3), 167-175.

Murray, N., Coy, P., Pater, J.L., *et al.* (1993) Importance of timing for thoracic irradiation in the combined modality treatment of limited-stage small-cell lung cancer: The National Cancer Institute of Canada Clinical Trials Group. *Journal of Clinical Oncology*, **11**, 336-344.

Pignon, J.P., Arriagada, R., Ihde, D.C., *et al.* (1992) A meta-analysis of thoracic radiotherapy for small-cell lung cancer. *New England Journal of Medicine*, **327** (23), 1618-1624.

PORT Meta-analysis Trialists Group (1998) *The Lancet*, **352** (9124), 257-263.

Price, P., Hoskin, P.J., Easton, D., Austin, D., Palmer, S.G., and Yarnold, J.R. (1986) Prospective randomised trial of single and multifraction radiotherapy schedules in the treatment of painful bony metastases. *Radiotherapy and Oncology*, **6**, 247-255.

Pritchard, R.S. and Anthony, S.P. (1996) Chemotherapy plus radiotherapy compared with radiotherapy alone in the treatment of locally advanced, unresectable, non-small-cell lung cancer: a meta-analysis *Annals of Internal Medicine*, **125**, 723-729.

Saunders, M.I., Dische, S., Barrett, A., *et al.* on behalf of the CHART Steering Committee (1999) Continuous, hyperfractionated, accelerated radiotherapy (CHART) versus conventional radiotherapy in non-small-cell lung cancer: Mature data from the Randomised Multicentre Trial. *Radiotherapy and Oncology*, **52**, 137-148.

Slotman, B.J. (2009) Prophylactic cranial irradiation in extensive disease small-cell lung cancer: short-term health-related quality of life and patient reported symptoms—results of an international phase III randomized controlled trial by the EORTC Radiation Oncology and Lung Cancer Groups. *Journal of Clinical Oncology*, **27** (1), 78-84.

Steenland, E., Leer, J.W., van Houwelingen, H., *et al.* (1999) The effect of a single fraction compared to multiple fractions on painful bone metastases: a global analysis of the Dutch Bone Metastasis Study. *Radiotherapy and Oncology*, **52**, 101-109.

Turrisi, A.T., Kim, K., Blum, R., *et al.* (1999) twice-daily compared with once-daily thoracic radiotherapy in limited small-cell lung cancer treated concurrently with cisplatin and etoposide. *New England Journal of Medicine*, **340**, 265–271.

Warde, P. and Payne, D. (1992) Does thoracic irradiation improve survival and local control in limited-stage small-cell carcinoma of the lung? A meta-analysis. *Journal of Clinical Oncology*, **10**, 890–895.

Chapter 5

Surgery for Lung Cancer

Neil Cartwright and Aman S. Coonar

Key points

- Surgery remains the gold standard treatment for lung cancer with curative intent.
- The operability and resectability of a lung cancer is best assessed by a thoracic surgeon as part of multidisciplinary team.
- Surgical procedures can be performed to clarify diagnosis and/or stage a tumour that is inaccessible to other techniques.
- Palliative surgical procedures play an important role in improving the quality of life in patients with advanced cancers.

Introduction

In the twentieth century thoracic surgery began to differentiate from general surgery. In part this came about because there was a drive to find treatments for suppurative lung diseases, particularly tuberculosis (TB). The specialty grew to include all the structures of the chest including the oesophagus, great vessels and heart. Because of the history of isolating many TB patients, and given the particular needs of such patients, the practice of thoracic surgery became concentrated in centres that were often free-standing and sometimes isolated. During this period, there were also important social changes in industrialised countries that led to better health for the community. The widespread availability of antibiotics contributed to this improvement. Unfortunately, during this time smoking also became popular and there was an increase in lung, head, neck and oesophageal cancers. Consequently, in the second half of the twentieth century surgical management of thoracic malignancy became common.

Lung Cancer: A Multidisciplinary Approach, First Edition. Edited by Alison Leary.
© 2012 Blackwell Publishing Ltd. Published 2012 by Blackwell Publishing Ltd.

In due course it became recognised that there was much variability in the availability of thoracic surgery and also that sometimes there were major differences in outcomes. Reasons for this included epidemiological factors, differences in the biology of the disease and, it seemed, differences in provision of services and specialists. Studies found the UK to be in the lower tiers of outcome within the industrialised nations. Research identified prolonged delays in referral and investigation prior to surgery. As a consequence, committed surgical and medical oncologists, other activists and politicians sought to address this in a number of initiatives, central to which was a view that all patients should be referred and investigated promptly and be discussed in a forum that included representatives of the specialist treatment providers, namely a surgeon and an oncologist and specialists in diagnostics and staging, such as a radiologist. This evolved into today's multidisciplinary team (MDT) and became a keystone in modern cancer management both in the UK and elsewhere.

In the UK, thoracic surgery is mostly performed by surgeons with a cardiothoracic surgical training. In other places, thoracic surgery is considered to be more of a subspecialty of general surgery. Some surgeons will have both a cardiac and thoracic surgical practice, whereas some will choose to focus exclusively on thoracic surgery.

More recently the trend of isolated centres has started to reverse. There are a number of reasons for this and they include the centralisation of specialist services, organisation of cancer networks, and the need for surgeons and related anaesthetic, nursing and other teams to have minimum numbers. Economies of scale and political factors have also been important. A further germane point is that modern medicine, driven by the desire for quality, is following a path of specialisation. Cardiothoracic surgery is no different and has differentiated into distinct subspecialties, such as adult cardiac surgery, paediatric cardiac surgery, general thoracic surgery and so on. However much surgeons enjoy variety in their work, the surgical community has recognised that often specialisation helps in the delivery of quality care. As a consequence, many major teaching hospitals in the modern world have units in which there are divisions of thoracic surgery.

UK lung cancer resection rates

Even though surgery is the best treatment for many patients, historically the UK had lower resection rates for lung cancer than many western European countries and North America. The reasons for this are multifactorial but were thought to relate to a lack of thoracic surgeons. There has been an increase in the numbers of such surgeons in the UK, but there continues to be an apparently important variation in resection rates in different parts of the UK. The reasons for this are not clear. One of the problems may be a bias against referring for surgery because the risk is perceived as too great. There is concern among UK surgeons that not all suitable patients are being referred. Consequently there is a proposal by some in the surgical community – including the present authors – that all patients with stage I–II, some patients with stage III and carefully selected patients with stage IV lung cancer be given the opportunity to meet a surgeon so that they can include that advice in their decision making. There are also efforts being made to manage risk-averse behaviour by surgeons or MDTs. Included in this there is the proposal that any patient who is turned down for surgery be offered the opportunity of a second surgical opinion.

Patient-centred decision making

In the modern NHS care is patient centred. While no surgeon would knowingly offer a treatment that they felt a patient could not tolerate, ultimately it is the patient who is to decide what for them is an acceptable risk and what they would accept in terms of post-treatment function. We feel that the relevant advice to assist the patient should include that from the surgeon. Consequently we consider that virtually all patients with resectable lung cancer should be given the opportunity to meet a surgeon along with other MDT members to assist their decision making process.

The role of the surgeon

Surgery plays an important role in the contemporary management of lung cancer and other thoracic malignancies with diagnostic, staging, curative or palliative procedures to offer. This chapter will discuss surgery and the role of the surgeon in the MDT as regards primary and secondary cancers of the lung. We recognise that there are many variations and one model will not fit all. This is a broad overview, some of which is evidence-based but also much of which reflects the senior author's current practice.

Referral to a surgeon

Patients may be referred to a surgeon at any stage of their disease pathway. Usually they are referred with a definite or suspected diagnosis of a cancer. In the UK, referral is often from a hospital physician or from the lung cancer MDT. In turn, the patient may have been referred from another specialist physician or directly from their general family practitioner. In many other countries, for example Canada or the USA, family practitioners may refer directly to thoracic surgeons, or a patient may purposefully seek them out. In the UK, it is recommended that if possible treatment be guided by the multidisciplinary team. When planning treatment it is important for the patient, professionals and commissioners of health care that this be timely, efficient and inclusive.

What can surgeons do?

Surgical practice varies in different parts of the world. In some jurisdictions almost all non-radiologically-guided invasive procedures will be undertaken by surgeons, ranging from all aspects of bronchoscopy to complex open surgery, including rarely even lung transplantation for lung cancer (De Perrot *et al.* 2004). In some places some simple radiological procedures are also undertaken by surgeons (Coonar *et al.* 2009a). In other places, such as the UK, considerable parts of the practice may be undertaken by interventionally minded non-surgeons. Each model has merits and limitations.

Role of the surgeon in the multidisciplinary team

In the UK, surgeons offer both diagnostic and therapeutic procedures to patients with known or suspected lung cancer. These procedures are described in more detail later in this chapter.

When there is uncertainty regarding diagnosis or stage, further biopsies can be obtained through procedures such as mediastinoscopy, mediastinotomy, video assisted thoracic surgery (VATS), or a mini-thoracotomy, In the treatment of lung cancer with curative intent, surgery remains an important choice for those patients who are deemed to be fit for surgery and have a resectable tumour. Surgery may also play a role in the palliation of patients with more advanced tumours, for whom procedures such as drainage of malignant pleural or pericardial effusions, control of intrathoracic sepsis or intrabronchial stenting can control symptoms and improve quality of life. These procedures are described in greater detail in the following sections.

Reaching decisions about surgery

In 2009 the classification and group staging systems for lung cancer were revised (Goldstraw *et al.* 2007; Groome *et al.* 2007; Postmus *et al.* 2007; Rami-Porta *et al.* 2007; Rusch *et al.* 2007). These have been developed by the International Association for the Study of Lung Cancer (IASLC) in cooperation with other organizations including the AJCC (American Joint Committee on Cancer) and the UICC (International Union Against Cancer) and are based on a much larger dataset than that used previously. The revised stage groups carry implications for treatment and prognosis and currently are among the best evidence on which to base advice to advise patients of their stage-specific outcome after surgery.

Reaching decisions about surgery: what factors need to be considered?

The surgeon needs to determine the correct operation (extent of planned surgery with consideration of anaesthetic requirements). If the aim of surgery is curative resection, the surgeon will determine to what extent a resection is required. In addition to the question whether the operation is technically possible, the patient must also be fit enough and have enough respiratory reserve to have an acceptable quality of life after the resection. Thus the surgeon will also assess the patient in terms of fitness for the planned surgery. Although an operation may be technically possible it is important that the morbidity of the operation does not outweigh the potential benefits. This will differ between cases, and sometimes the advice of an MDT can be valuable. The patient's own views are essential in determining what is acceptable.

What is the extent of surgery required, and what are the anaesthetic considerations?

These considerations will depend of the goals of the surgery. For example, palliation of a pleural effusion by means of drain insertion under local anaesthesia and sedation followed by talc poudrage may be quite appropriate for a frail patient, whereas an extensive pleurectomy with general anaesthesia and epidural regional anaesthesia may be offered to a fitter patient with the goals of both palliating the effusion and reducing tumour bulk. The latter operation may carry excessive risks to the frail patient, whose life expectancy and quality of life may also be reduced due to other medical problems.

Resectability

Resectability is a judgement on the possibility of complete surgical resection of a cancer (Lim *et al.* 2010). This is dependent on the cell type, anatomical position, extent of local invasion and distant spread. The standard operations are a lobectomy, bilobectomy or pneumonectomy, and a lymph node dissection. Under some circumstances a smaller resection (such as an anatomical segmentectomy or a non-anatomical wedge resection) can be justified. This may be appropriate for a low-grade tumour such as a typical carcinoid or in cases of poor lung function. Variations of anatomical resections can be performed, which include resection and reconstruction of the airway or pulmonary artery. These are known as 'sleeve resections'.

It is the surgeon's role to assess whether resection can be performed with an adequate margin from the tumour without significant or unacceptable damage to other important structures. Incomplete resections are associated with poorer outcomes in the form of higher rates of local recurrence and reduced survival (Chamogeorgakis *et al.* 2009). Occasionally this is the best option for a patient, particularly in the context of multimodality treatment.

Following surgery, the completeness of a resection is described using the 'R' classification. This is shown in Box 5.1.

> ## Box 5.1   The 'R' classification
>
> **R   Definition**
> R0   Complete microscopic and macroscopic resection
> R1   Residual microscopic disease
> R2   Residual macroscopic disease

The aim of surgery with curative intent is to leave no residual disease (R0). In cases of incomplete resection, the MDT will usually have a helpful discussion regarding the merits of further surgery or intervention, local radiotherapy or chemotherapy.

Comment

There are variable approaches to the surgical management of lung cancer. Historically, and influenced by the poorer survival of lung cancer patients, the general approach was often more conservative. However, work by many groups worldwide has led to improved outcomes and current approaches tend to be much more aggressive.

The concept of 'benefit of the doubt'

It is not unusual for there to be uncertainty about the stage of a patient's tumour and, if appropriate, the MDT may agree on a lower stage. A relatively common example of this is the situation of two (or occasionally more) nodules. After staging investigations, if the pattern could be explained by two (or more) primaries rather than metastatic spread many MDTs would consider erring toward the former position, even though the possibility of one being a metastasis from the other could not be completely discounted. Accepting a lower stage justifies offering a more radical treatment. Adopting a favourable position despite uncertainty is described as 'benefit of the doubt'. This aggressive approach arises from the uncertainty in being able to reliably predict which patients will benefit *most* from a given treatment and who will not. Another relatively common example may be that of a proximal tumour for which the margin can only be confirmed at or after the time of surgery when detailed pathological examination has been performed. Applying further the logic of this argument means that to offer a patient the best chance of survival requires being able to offer the most aggressive treatment, bearing in mind their wishes, co-morbidities, overall fitness and the stage of the tumour.

Fitness for surgery or 'operability'

Fitness for surgery is related to the extent of the proposed surgery and the overall capacity of the patient to withstand the requirements of surgery, general anaesthesia and a return to a level of function that is acceptable to them. The first step is for an experienced clinician to form an opinion regarding fitness for surgery. The value of a clear history and clinical assessment, for example by walking with the patient on the ward or up a flight of stairs, can be very important as it sums several different factors including overall strength, coordination and motivation. In such cases, poor lung function tests may be given less significance in patients with a preserved exercise and performance capacity.

Case study: Left pneumonectomy in a patient with impaired lung function

A 66-year-old 'fit' man
Distal LMB/LUL NSCLC
Emphysema
Smoker
$FEV_1 = 2 = 64.9\%$
$FVC = 4.3 = 108\%$
$TLCO = 41\%$

$TLC = 8 L = 117\%$
$RV = 3.79 l = 151.6\%$
Desaturated; S_aO_2 fell from 97% to 80% at 520 m
Echocardiogram PAP 42 mmHg at rest
Ventilation 65% right
Perfusion 65% right

Abbreviations: FEV_1, forced expiratory volume in 1 second; FVC, forced vital capacity; RV, residual volume; TLCO, transfer factor for carbon monoxide (CO) in the lung; VA, alveolar ventilation.

The patient was still working in a physically demanding job, very motivated for radical treatment and willing to accept a reduced level of function. Postoperatively this patient was found to have a T2 N1 completely resected cancer. He was discharged after 8 days, and was disease free and with good performance status >2 years after surgery he has returned to work.

Figure 5.1 is a preoperative CXR showing loss of clear left heart border. Figure 5.2 shows the distal left main bronchus/left upper lobe tumour with

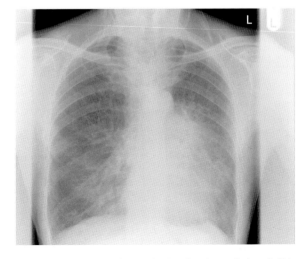

Fig. 5.1 Preoperative chest radiograph showing loss of clear left heart border.

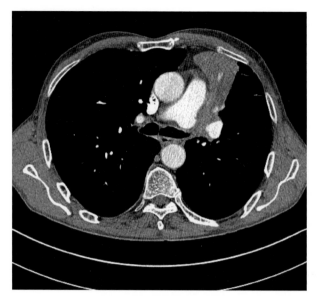

Fig. 5.2 CT of the distal left main bronchus /left upper lobe tumour with collapse of the lingula. Probable proximal left pulmonary artery involvement.

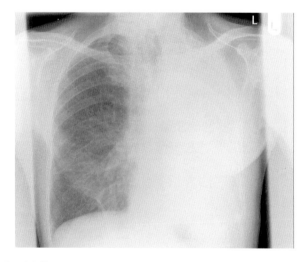

Fig. 5.3 Post left pneumonectomy.

collapse of the lingula and probable proximal left pulmonary artery involvement. Figure 5.3 shows the patient post left pneumonectomy.

In such cases the MDT approach to assessing the preoperative functional status of a patient can be valuable. Guidelines have been produced to help guide assessment for surgery. The guidelines produced in 2001 by the British Thoracic Society (BTS) (British Thoracic Society 2001)

Table 5.1 ACCP guidelines for assessment of lung function in patients considered for surgery (Colice *et al.* 2007).

1. It is recommended that patients with lung cancer be assessed for curative surgical resection by a multidisciplinary team, which includes a thoracic surgeon specializing in lung cancer, a medical oncologist, a radiation oncologist, and a pulmonologist (chest physician).

2. It is recommended that patients with lung cancer not be denied lung resection surgery on the grounds of age alone.

3. It is recommended that patients with lung cancer who are being evaluated for surgery and have major factors for increased perioperative cardiovascular risk have a preoperative cardiologic evaluation.

4. In patients being considered for lung cancer resection, spirometry is recommended. If the FEV_1 is >80% predicted or >2 L and there is no evidence of either undue dyspnoea on exertion or interstitial lung disease, the patient is suitable for resection including pneumonectomy without a further physiological evaluation. If the FEV_1 is >1.5 L and there is no evidence of either undue dyspnoea on exertion or interstitial lung disease, the patient is suitable for a lobectomy without further physiological evaluation.

5. In patients being considered for lung cancer resection, if there is evidence of either undue dyspnoea on exertion or interstitial lung disease, even though the FEV_1 might be adequate, measuring TLCO is recommended.

6. In patients being considered for lung cancer resection, if either the FEV_1 or TLCO are <80% predicted, it is recommended that postoperative lung function be predicted through additional testing.

7. In patients with lung cancer who are being considered for surgery, either an FEV_1 of < 0%ppo or a TLCO of <40%ppo indicates an increased risk for perioperative death and cardiopulmonary complications with standard lung resection. It is recommended that these patients undergo exercise testing preoperatively.

8. In patients with lung cancer who are being considered for surgery, either a product of %ppo FEV_1 and %ppo TLCO of <1650%ppo or an FEV_1 of <30%ppo indicates an increased risk for perioperative death and cardiopulmonary complications with standard lung resection. It is recommended that these patients should be counselled about non-standard surgery and non-operative treatment options for their lung cancer.

9. In patients with lung cancer being considered for surgery, a $\dot{v}O_2$max of <10 mL/kg/min indicates an increased risk for perioperative death and cardiopulmonary complications with standard lung resection. These patients should be counselled about non-standard surgery and non-operative treatment options for their lung cancer.

10. Patients with lung cancer being considered for surgery who have a $\dot{v}O_2$max of <15 mL/kg/min and both an FEV_1 and a TLCO of <40%ppo are at an increased risk for perioperative death and cardiopulmonary complications with standard lung resection. It is recommended that these patients be counselled about non-standard surgery and non-operative treatment options for their lung cancer.

(Continued)

Table 5.1 (*Continued*)

11. Patients with lung cancer being considered for surgery who walk <25 shuttles on two shuttle walks or less than one flight of stairs are at increased risk for perioperative death and cardiopulmonary complications with standard lung resection. These patients should be counselled about non-standard surgery and non-operative treatment options for their lung cancer.

12. In patients with lung cancer who are being considered for surgery, a P_aCO_2 of >45 mmHg is not an independent risk factor for increased perioperative complications. However, it is recommended that these patients undergo further physiological testing.

13. In patients with lung cancer who are being considered for surgery, an S_aO_2 of <90% indicates an increased risk for perioperative complications with standard lung resection. It is recommended that these patients undergo further physiological testing.

14. In patients with very poor lung function and a lung cancer in an area of upper lobe emphysema, it is recommended that combined LVRS and lung cancer resection be considered if both the FEV_1 and the TLCO are >20% predicted.

15. It is recommended that all patients with lung cancer be counselled regarding smoking cessation.

were considered to be fairly conservative and most surgeons were more aggressive. More recent guidelines include those published by the American College of Chest Physicians (ACCP) in 2007 (Colice *et al.* 2007), joint task forces of the European Respiratory Society and European Society of Thoracic Surgeons (Brunelli *et al.* 2009), and the British Thoracic Society and Society of Cardiothoracic Surgeons (SCTS). Although they differ in some respects, they are generally similar, but there is controversy between the advocates of different assessment algorithms. Clinically well patients with acceptable lung function ($FEV_1 > 1.5$–2 L, and TLCO > 40%) are generally considered to be low risk. In patients with co-morbidity or impaired lung function there is an emphasis on correction or control of co-morbidities (for example, urgent revascularisation for significant coronary artery disease) and an estimation of predicted postoperative lung function. This allows the patient to be given both a rough estimate of mortality and also quality of life postoperatively. In the recent BTS/SCTS guidelines a ppoFEV1 or ppoTLCO of <40% are used to suggest a moderate to high risk of post-treatment dyspnoea.

Comment

It should be recognised that these are *only* guidelines and some surgeons and MDTs, including the author, will offer surgery to patients who do not fulfil the guideline criteria and still achieve good results. Indeed, many thoracic surgeons consider the guidelines to be over-conservative in assessing the suitability of patients for lung resection. It is thus not surprising that the assessment of fitness for surgery is an area of active debate and research (Brunelli 2008).

The formal assessment of lung function

Spirometry with estimations of lung volumes (FEV_1, FVC, FRC, RV, TLC), measures of gas transfer (TLCO and KCO (KCO = TLCO/VA)) and physiological tests (exercise oximetry or metabolic oxygen consumption) currently form the basis of objective evaluation of fitness for surgery. Algorithms to assist in the selection of patients for surgery are available. As mentioned above, cut-offs to determine when surgery is unacceptable are not well defined.

The role of FEV_1 in determining operability for lung resection

Assessment of pulmonary function is thought to have some importance. Some guidelines referred to a meta-analysis of three large series in the 1970s that demonstrated that a preoperative forced expiratory volume in 1 second (FEV_1) of >1.5 L for lobectomy or >2.0 L for pneumonectomy carried a mortality rate of less than 5% (Boushy *et al*. 1971; Miller 1993). As this appeared to be an acceptable level of risk, it provided guidance for a generation of thoracic surgeons, but limitations in the data have always been recognised. The data was not well controlled and extrapolating by age, height or gender was difficult. In addition, other investigation suggest it to be over-conservative (Olsen *et al*. 1974; Pate *et al*. 1996).

For patients who do not meet the normal lung function requirements for lobectomy or pneumonectomy, further assessment of lung function may be helpful. A ventilation-perfusion scan provides additional information on the relative contribution of the regions of the lungs and an estimate can be made of the relative contributions of different bronchopulmonary lung segments. An estimate of postoperative lung function can also be made by calculating how many of the 19 segments of the lung will be removed, and allows for the loss of functional and non-functional segments (Equation 5.1).

Equation 5.1 (modified from the BTS guidelines)

Expected post-operative FEV1 = pre-operative FEV1 × (19-segments to be removed)/19

a modification is used if segments are already not working.

Table 5.2 Preoperative assessment of cardiac function and risk. Adapted from BTS guidelines on cardiological assessment for patients being considered for pulmonary resections

1. All patients for lung resection should have a preoperative ECG.

2. All patients with an audible cardiac murmur should have an echocardiogram.

3. Patients who have had a myocardial infarction should normally not be operated on for lung resection within 6 weeks.

4. Any patient who has had a myocardial infarction within 6 months and is being assessed for thoracic surgery should have a cardiology opinion.

5. Patients who have had coronary artery bypass surgery should not be precluded from having lung resection. They should be assessed as for other patients with possible cardiac risk factors.

6. The guidelines from the American College of Cardiology and the American Heart Association should be used as a basis for assessing the perioperative cardiovascular risk of patients undergoing lung resection.

The patient with emphysema

However, using Equation 5.1 becomes relatively unreliable in patients with significant emphysema. In this group, removal of poorly functioning parts of the lung may be associated with a *smaller then expected deterioration or even an improvement* in lung function, which is known as the 'lung volume reduction surgery' (LVRS) effect. LVRS is thought to work by two main mechanisms: firstly by improving ventilation-perfusion matching in the remaining lung, and secondly by reducing hyperinflation and in so doing reducing the work of breathing.

For those patients deemed at high risk, a full discussion between members of the multidisciplinary team often helps to decide which treatment option may be best. In such patients limited, resections including wedge resections, anatomical segmentectomy or sleeve resections, or an entirely different approach involving a non-surgical treatment such as radiotherapy or radiofrequency ablation (RFA) (Lencioni *et al.* 2008) may be most suitable.

Cardiovascular risks

Particular attention should also be paid to cardiovascular risk in patients with lung cancer, as smoking is a common risk factor for both diseases. Both the ACCP and BTS have advice on the preoperative assessment of cardiac function and risk. This is summarised in Table 5.2.

Advising patients on the risks of surgery

Risk stratification is not as highly developed in thoracic surgery as in its partner cardiac surgery, in which risk models have become sophisticated and widely used. Different models are under development (e.g. Thoracoscore) and there is a search for a consensus (Berrisford *et al.* 2005; Falcoz *et al.* 2007; Brunelli *et al.* 2008; Ferguson *et al.* 2008; Wright *et al.* 2008). Although there are differences, fairly consistent findings were that risk increased with age and with level of dyspnoea and whether a pneumonectomy was performed. Adverse outcome has been associated with other factors such as diabetes, low body mass index and recent cardiac problems.

In the UK, the Society of Cardiothoracic Surgeons requests information from all units engaged in thoracic surgery. In 2008 the first national thoracic surgery activity and outcomes report was published (SCTS 2008). This includes data to 2005 and from this a number of comments can be made. Firstly, the outcomes from thoracic surgery units are satisfactory with respect to in-hospital mortality. Reasonable approximate mortality estimates without risk stratification are about 2–3% for lobectomy and about 6–8% after pneumonectomy. It is generally agreed that a right pneumonectomy carries a greater risk than a left-sided procedure. The mortality after a wedge resection is also about 2%. Although this is a lesser resection, a relatively larger proportion of these patients will have other co-morbidities that seem to place them at higher risk. The rate of exploratory thoracotomy not proceeding to lung resection (also known as the 'open and close' rate) is about 5%.

Partly owing to the controversies in risk-scoring for thoracic surgery, in the authors' unit an additional approach to reducing risk has been taken. Using a model adopted from industry, all postsurgical deaths undergo detailed pathway analysis followed by open and constructive team discussion with the purpose of identifying steps that, if modified, might have led to a more favourable outcome. In our unit a review of all patients who underwent thoracic surgery over 5 years between 2006 and 2010 was undertaken and we found the mortality to be <0.8%. In only 0.2% were steps identified that might have led to a different outcome. By applying those system modifications, it is hoped that mortality and other complications may be further minimised (Ali *et al.* 2011).

Papworth Thoracic Surgery Unit strategies to reduce risk

- Airway toilet
  Liberal use of surgeon-performed awake flexible bronchoscopy for airway toilet.
- Minimising aspiration
  Low threshold to place patients 'nil by mouth' until strong cough is established. Nasogastric or parenteral feeding as required.
- Systematic use of venous thromboembolism prophylaxis.
- Systematic use of peptic ulcer prophylaxis.
- Systematic use of central venous catheter during major anatomical lung resection unless specifically agreed between consultant surgeon and anaesthetist.

> **Box 5.2   Methods of obtaining a pathological diagnosis – those in bold type are the specific remit of thoracic surgeons but other techniques may also be performed by surgeons**
>
> Sputum examination
> Pleural fluid aspiration (often radiologically guided) and examination
> Percutaneous needle biopsy (often radiologically guided)
> Bronchoscopy with washing, brushings or biopsy
> Endobronchial or endo-oesophageal ultrasound-guided needle aspiration
> **Mediastinoscopy**
> **Mediastinotomy**
> **Minimally invasive surgical techniques**
> **Open surgery**

Surgery for cancers of the lung

Cancers of the lung may be regarded as primary tumours arising in the lung or secondary tumours (metastases) that have spread to the lung. Primary lung cancer is further classified according to cell type. Although these classifications oversimplify, they are useful for clinical decision making, as there are important differences in the current management of small-cell lung cancer (SCLC) (Samson *et al.* 2007; Simon and Turrisi 2007) and non-small-cell lung cancer (NSCLC). Only a small proportion of SCLC that presents early (T1-2 N0 M0) may be suitable for surgery (Wadell and Shepherd 2004). In order to better establish the role of surgery in SCLC, efforts are being made to offer surgery as part of trials. Sometimes carcinoid tumours and bronchoalveolar cancer are managed differently. Comments regarding the management of these subtypes of lung cancer are made later.

Once a patient presents with a suspicion of malignancy, attention is directed towards diagnosis and staging.

Invasive biopsy and staging

In some cases a strong clinical suspicion of cancer will be enough to merit surgery. However, for most patients a firm cytological or histological diagnosis is preferred. Box 5.2 outlines methods for obtaining pathological diagnosis and Boxes 5.3–5.6 elaborate on some of these.

Pathological diagnosis at the time of definitive surgery ('frozen section')

If biopsy is required at the time of planned definitive surgery, this would normally be in the context of there being strong clinical evidence for malignancy. It is important to recognise that a rapid pathological diagnosis

> ## Box 5.3   Mediastinoscopy
>
> Day-case.
> General anaesthesia.
> Single-lumen endotracheal tube with two-lung ventilation.
> Local anaesthetic infiltration to surgical site.
> 2–4 cm skin crease collar incision.
> Dissection to the pretracheal plane with biopsies – usually of stations 2R, 4R, (right paratracheal) 2L, 4L (left paratracheal) and 7 (subcarinal) lymph nodes.
> Performed either under direct vision through a mediastinoscope and increasingly by the use of a video-mediastinoscope, which allows the operation to be performed by viewing the operation on a screen.
> Wound closure with dissolving suture material.
>
> *General complications of surgery*
> Pain, infection, bleeding.
>
> *Specific complications*
> Conversion to thoracotomy or sternotomy (<1%), pneumothorax (<5%).
> Mortality (<0.1%).
>
> *Follow-up*
> Usually follow-up by the surgeon is not needed, though some surgeons would prefer to review the patient to be satisfied that the wound is satisfactory.
>
> *Comment*
> Most patients recover quickly and manage with either no analgesia or paracetamol. If the patient does not require further surgery, many surgeons would be agreeable to follow-up by the referring physician alone, though individual practices will differ.

obtained at the time of operation is limited compared with one obtained prior to definitive surgery. Most modern guidelines encourage preoperative histological diagnosis.

With technological advances, bronchoscopic biopsy may now be guided by immunofluorescence to illuminate abnormal areas of epithelium, or ultrasound (endo-oesophageal or endobronchial) to guide lymph node biopsy (Yasufuku *et al.* 2007; Rintoul *et al.* 2009).

Lung resections with curative intent

The history of the 'T' descriptor is that T1–3 were considered to be resectable by 'standard' techniques, whereas T4 tumours, classified because of involvement of vital structures, were considered unresectable by 'standard' techniques. T4 tumours include cancers with mediastinal, vertebral, cardiac,

Box 5.4   Mediastinotomy

This is usually left-sided but sometimes is performed on the right side.
Day-case or overnight stay.
General anaesthesia.
Local anaesthetic infiltration to surgical site.
Double-lumen tube with isolation of the ipsilateral lung to improve exposure can be helpful. Some surgeons would accept a single-lumen tube with intermittent apnoea.
3–6 cm transverse incision over the second intercostal space, just lateral to the internal mammary pedicle. A section of second costal cartilage or rib can be excised to improve exposure.
The path of dissection can be either medial to the mediastinal pleura or intrapleural. Biopsies – usually of station 5 (subaortic) and 6 (para-aortic) lymph nodes can be obtained.
Performed either under direct vision through a mediastinoscope and increasingly by the use of a video-mediastinoscope. If the pleural space has been entered, air can be evacuated and a chest tube removed at the end of the case or later.
Wound closure with dissolving suture material.

General complications of surgery
Pain, infection, bleeding, scar

Specific complications or warnings
Chest tube. Conversion to thoracotomy or sternotomy (<1%).
Mortality (<0.1%).
Long term pain (rare)

Follow-up
Many surgeons will be comfortable with follow-up by the referring physician only, though some surgeons would prefer to review the patient once to be satisfied that the wound is satisfactory.

oesophageal, tracheal or carinal involvement. By the use of 'non-standard' surgical techniques, resection may be possible with acceptable results. TNM staging has progressed and the 7th edition published in 2010 is discussed elsewhere.

Operations include sublobar resections, lobectomy, bilobectomy and pneumonectomy and airway resections. In general, the greater the resection the lower is the recurrence rate. However, a surgical decision is also guided by patient fitness. In order to preserve lung function, sublobar resections such as a segmentectomy or non-anatomical wedge resection can be performed. This may be indicated if the patient has relatively poor lung function or if there are synchronous lesions and it becomes more important

Box 5.5 Video-assisted thoracic surgery (VATS) with biopsies

Usually 1-3 night stay.

General anaesthesia.

Double-lumen endotracheal tube with ipsilateral lung isolation to improve exposure.

Local anaesthetic infiltration to surgical sites.

Typically 1-3 incisions (5-3 cm).

Entry to the intrapleural space and identification of target lymph nodes or sites of concern. Particularly helpful for biopsy of the pleura, station 5 (subaortic) and 6 (para-aortic), 8 (para-oesophageal), 9 (inferior pulmonary ligament) lymph nodes, anterior mediastinum and lung biopsy. Station 7 can also be accessed.

Wound closure with dissolving suture material and removable suture for the drain.

General complications of surgery
Pain, infection, bleeding, scar.

Specific complications
Conversion to open thoracotomy (<1%).
Mortality (<0.1%)
Long term pain (uncommon).

Follow-up
Many surgeons prefer to review patients who have had VATS surgery.

Box 5.6 Mini/limited thoracotomy and biopsy

A small incision (mini/limited thoracotomy), which may be video-assisted, can be undertaken or this may be performed at the time of planned definitive surgery. A larger incision (full thoracotomy) can be justified when it is very important to obtain excellent control, for example biopsying a node on a vascular structure or to obtain a better impression of resectability. The incision can be muscle-sparing.

---

to preserve lung function. As mentioned elsewhere, the recurrence rate may be greater with a sublobar resection.

The majority of lung resections are performed through a thoracotomy. As experience with video-assisted thoracic surgery (VATS) has increased, more centres now offer lobectomy for selected patients as a minimally invasive procedure.

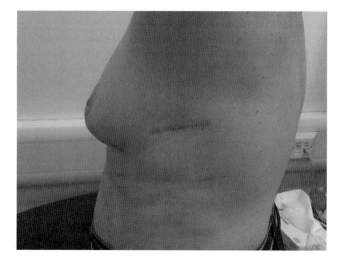

Fig. 5.4 Side view of a patient approximately 4 weeks after VATS lobectomy and lymph node dissection. The 9-cm incision is used both to operate through and also to extract the lobe through. Two other approximately 1.5-cm incisions are also visible. One is used for the telescope and the other for an instrument.

VATS lung resections

According to the 2008 SCTS thoracic surgery report (SCTS 2008) in the UK only about 2% of lobectomies were performed by VATS. This reflects a number of considerations including technical demands, additional time that may be required, and learning curve for the whole team, but also very importantly concern as to the completeness of resection or adequacy of lymph node dissection. Proving equivalence or superiority of an open technique lung resection over a minimal access one is very difficult, and good comparisons in sizeable numbers have not been performed. In any case, until VATS lobectomies can be generalised more widely it seems likely that the majority of lung resections will continue to be performed as fully open procedures. There are important advances in the development of VATS equipment, and this may encourage the take-up of this technique.

A greater proportion of sublobar resections are performed by VATS. The majority of these are non-anatomical wedge resections

Figure 5.4 shows a side view of a patient approximately 4 weeks after VATS lobectomy and lymph node dissection undertaken at Papworth Hospital by the senior author. The approximately 9 cm (3.5 inch) utility incision was used both to operate through and to extract the lobe (about half the lung volume) without damaging it or the tumour mass. Two other approximately 1.5 cm incisions are also visible. One is used for the telescope and the other for an instrument. In some cases smaller utility incisions are used, but many surgeons find extraction of the lobe difficult (particularly if

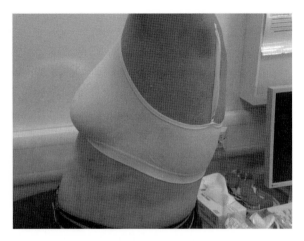

Fig. 5.5   The scar is cosmetic and can be hidden easily under clothing. Only a single port site scar is now visible. There is a very good range of shoulder movement.

the tumour is >2–3 cm) without running the risk of excessive lung or even tumour contusion, hence use of a utility incision of around 8–9 cm.

Figure 5.5 shows that the scar can be hidden easily under clothing. Only a single port site scar is now visible. There is a very good range of shoulder movement.

T3/T4 resections when an important structure is involved

Surgery may also be considered for patients with T3 or T4 tumours. Resection of these tumours usually involves en-bloc resection of the invaded structure such as part of the chest wall, diaphragm or pericardium. The outcome in these cases can be favourable providing a satisfactory margin is obtained. Following such a resection it may be necessary to reconstruct a defect to prevent problems such as herniation of intrathoracic contents or mechanical compromise causing ventilatory failure. This can be achieved by use of biological or synthetic materials. Novel techniques are under development and include, for example, the use of titanium implants bridging portions of resected ribs (Coonar *et al.* 2009b). This may have benefits with respect to maintaining ventilatory function (Coonar *et al.* 2011). Figure 5.6 shows a preoperative CT scan. In this patient with a low preoperative FEV_1, there is large tumour mass in the right chest involving the diaphragm. Figure 5.7 is the postoperative CT scan following resection by bilobectomy and diaphragm. The diaphragm has been reconstructed with an ePTFE sheet. The mass was a completely resected T3 N0 squamous cell carcinoma.

T4 tumours were classified as such because they invade 'vital structures' including the heart, great vessels, trachea, oesophagus or vertebral

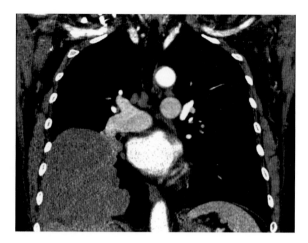

Fig. 5.6 Preoperative CT scan showing large tumour mass in right chest involving the diaphragm.

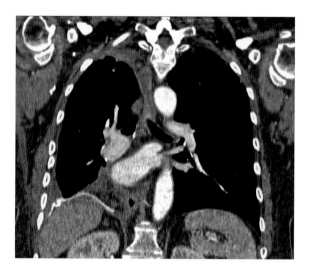

Fig. 5.7 Postoperative CT scan following resection by bilobectomy and diaphragm reconstruction. The diaphragm has been reconstructed with an ePTFE sheet. The mass was a completely resected T3N0 squamous cell carcinoma.

column. Some T4 tumours may be resectable using strategies such as cardiopulmonary bypass or with spinal stabilisation to allow vertebrectomy en-bloc with the tumour. In the case of Pancoast (superior sulcus) tumours, some teams will use neo-adjuvant treatment to downstage the tumours (Fischer *et al.* 2008) with the intention of improving the chance of complete resection. Some other groups prefer not to use preoperative induction treatment and also achieve satisfactory outcomes (Fadel *et al.* 2002).

Open surgery

The incision

The usual approach for an anatomical lung resection is a unilateral thoracotomy. The commonest incision is described as posterolateral and involves incision of the latissimus dorsi muscle and either reflection or division of the serratus anterior muscle. Other options include an anterior or anterolateral thoracotomy and muscle-splitting or muscle-sparing incisions. Additional approaches include midline sternotomy and bilateral thoracotomy (clamshell incision).

Pain control after thoracotomy

Epidural, extrapleural, paravertebral or intercostal nerve blocks

The surgeon and anaesthetist usually identify and agree on an optimal method of perioperative pain control. This usually also involves some form of local or regional anaesthesia as well as medication with paracetamol, non-steroidal anti-inflammatory drugs, gabapentin and opioids. The latter are often given in the form of patient-controlled analgesia (PCA) in which the patient can press a demand button and receive medication up to pre-set limits. It is usually possible to establish the patient on oral analgesia alone within 3–4 days post-operatively (Hughes and MacKay 2008).

There is increasing evidence that extrapleural regional anaesthesia is equivalent to epidural anaesthesia and may have fewer and less severe side effects (Joshi *et al.* 2008). The differences between paravertebral and extrapleural anaesthesia are marginal as they both rely on a regional intercostal nerve block by delivery into the extrapleural plane close to the vertebral column. The surgeon may also choose surgical techniques that are thought to reduce postoperative pain (Cerfolio *et al.* 2005). This can involve protection of the intercostal pedicle.

Unfortunately, a small number of people will experience long-term pain or paraesthesia associated with their wound. It is hard to predict who will be so effected and it is very important to warn people of this well-recognised complication (Katz *et al.* 1996). The input of a pain specialist can be useful at this late stage.

Recovery, discharge and mobilisation after thoracotomy

Most patients will be discharged within 1 week following a thoracotomy and will increase their activity. At around 6 weeks post surgery some patients will still be taking oral analgesia. Patients who have had VATS lung resections usually leave hospital in a slightly shorter time.

The role of adjuvant treatment in NSCLC

Adjuvant treatment after lung resection is influenced by a number of factors including the postoperative stage of the cancer, cell type, fitness of the patient, the use of neo-adjuvant treatment and the wishes of the patient. These factors are discussed in the MDT and appropriate advice is given.

Several studies have examined the role of postoperative chemotherapy, radiotherapy and chemoradiotherapy regimes. The results have been somewhat mixed. The results of systematic reviews provide evidence for current practice. A recent expert review recommended that adjuvant cisplatin-based chemotherapy be used routinely in patients with resected stages IIA, IIB and IIIA disease. Overall results of subset analyses for patient populations with stage IB disease were not significant, and thus adjuvant chemotherapy in stage IB disease was not recommended for routine use. Patients with stage IA NSCLC are not advised to have adjuvant therapy. Evidence from RCTs demonstrates a survival detriment for adjuvant radiotherapy with limited evidence for a reduction in local recurrence. Adjuvant radiation therapy appears detrimental to survival in stages IB and II, and may possibly confer a modest benefit in stage IIIA (Pisters et al. 2007).

Special situations

N2 disease

Preoperative identification of the involvement of N2 nodes is associated with a poorer prognosis, assumed to be because the identification of this level of nodal involvement implies more extensive spread. The management of N2 disease is controversial and variable (Robinson et al. 2007). Partly this is because there is much variation in what constitutes N2-positive disease varying from single-station microscopic disease at the first N2 station from the tumour discovered incidentally on postoperative pathological examination, to bulky multistation N2 disease evident preoperatively. Depending on the extent of N2 disease and the fitness of the patient, some groups advocate up-front surgery followed by chemoradiotherapy, whereas others follow an induction approach followed by surgery (see Chapters 3 & 4).

N2 disease has been classified into four subgroups; these are shown in Table 5.3.

IIIA1-2 disease

For patients with NSCLC who have incidental (occult) N2 disease (IIIA2) found at surgical resection and in whom complete resection of the lymph nodes and primary tumour is technically possible, the ACCP guidelines advise completion of the planned lung resection and mediastinal lymphadenectomy.

Qualifying this is the recognition that if a complex or higher-morbidity resection is required, such as a right pneumonectomy in a frail patient, then it could be reasonable not to proceed with the resection and to offer chemoradiotherapy.

Table 5.3 Subsets of stage IIIA(N2).

Subset Description

IIIA$_1$ Incidental nodal metastases found on final pathology examination of the resection specimen

IIIA$_2$ Nodal (single station) metastases recognized intraoperatively

IIIA$_3$ Nodal metastases (single or multiple station) recognized by pre-thoracotomy staging (mediastinoscopy, other nodal biopsy, or PET scan)

IIIA$_4$ Bulky or fixed multistation N2 disease

Adapted from Robinson *et al.* (2007).

Other groups have advocated closing the patient, offering induction treatment and then going onto resection (Russell and Ferguson 2007).

IIIA$_3$ disease

This is the group in whom N2 disease is diagnosed preoperatively, and is distinguished from IIIA$_4$ in which the disease is bulky and/or fixed. Again there is a wide range of opinion as to management. The data is mixed and high-quality clinical trials with large numbers are not available. Some surgeons and MDTs take the view that this represents advanced disease and a non-surgical approach is warranted. Other groups advise radical surgery involving lung resection and lymphadenectomy followed by adjuvant treatment, and others recommend induction treatment followed by surgery.

The current ACCP guidelines advise that in NSCLC patients with N2 disease identified preoperatively (IIIA$_3$), surgery should be offered as part of a clinical trial of induction or adjuvant therapy. In some series a high mortality rate has been noted after induction treatment followed by pneumonectomy, and therefore this is not advised in the ACCP guidelines. Despite this position there are also many survivors following such an approach.

Outcomes

There is a wide variation in survival rates. Presumably this reflects the complexity of identifying suitable patients, different regimes and differences in surgery. Five-year survival rates up to 40–50% have been reported in case series of patients having induction treatment followed by surgery.

Surgical management of metastases

The finding of distant metastasis is usually a contraindication to surgery for NSCLC. However, there are particular instances in which, if the metastatic disease can be controlled, long-term survival may be achieved with concurrent lung resection. Notable successes have been achieved in patients with adrenal and cerebral metastases. In these cases a combination of local control with surgery or radiotherapy, systemic chemotherapy and definitive surgical resection of the primary has yielded some long-term survivors. It is important to recognise that only a small number of patients can be treated successfully in this way.

With respect to adrenal metastases, a recent review suggested 5-year survival rates of approximately 25% (Tanvetyanon *et al.* 2008) after adrenalectomy, surgical resection and chemotherapy/radiotherapy.

The brain is another common site of metastasis. A small number of patients have had resection or radiotherapy of single brain metastasis or even of a few. Five-year survival rates of up to about 20% have also been reported (Flannery *et al.* 2005). Recent practice guidelines support the resection or ablation of brain metastases in highly selected patients as part of the management of their lung cancer (Mintz *et al.* 2007; Shen *et al.* 2007).

Recurrent disease

Surgery can be considered in cases of recurrent disease after previous surgery or after chemoradiotherapy. In these cases re-staging is performed and then treatment is offered on an individual basis. In these cases it is difficult to advise on prognosis. Many surgeons will re-stage the tumour as if it were a completely new tumour. However in the case of previous adverse features such as previous N2+ or more distant disease, the potential benefits of further surgery have to be somewhat tempered. In addition, the surgical risks can be greater as a result of the previous treatment, for example adhesions.

Palliative surgical procedures

Surgery can play a role in the palliation of patients with advanced lung cancer when complete resection is not possible. A key issue is to balance the risks of an intervention against its benefits. Measuring benefit in such patients is difficult, particularly when mortality is a poor outcome measure.

Possible indications for surgery:

- Bleeding
- Sepsis
- Pleural effusion/breathlessness
- Pneumothorax
- Pain
- Chest wall invasion

Some examples of surgical intervention are discussed. Surgery may be indicated for uncontrolled intrathoracic sepsis. For instance, resection of an abscess or drainage of an empyema may improve quality of life.

Pleural effusions are a common problem for patients with cancer. These can cause breathlessness, and some oncologists would prefer these to be treated before chemotherapy. A pleural effusion can be handled in different ways. Strategies include observation, aspiration or drainage with variously sized tubes, intermittent drainage with a tunnelled pleural catheter, or handling with thoracoscopy/thoracotomy. If the lung expands well after drainage of the effusion, pleurodesis may be possible by pleural abrasion, pleurectomy, or sterile

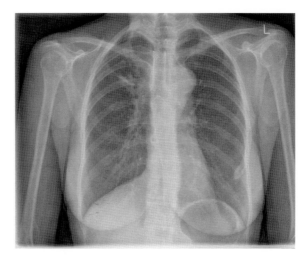

Fig. 5.8   Chest radiograph showing Y-stent in trachea opening into R + L main bronchi.

talc or other agents. If the lung remains trapped, repeated aspiration or a long-term tunnelled drain may be more effective in control of the pleural effusion.

Similarly, a pericardial effusion may cause symptoms as cardiac filling becomes restricted. Drainage through a pericardial window or by a simple drain may be effective. Symptoms of breathlessness may also be due to obstruction of an airway by direct invasion or by a pressure effect. This also puts the distal lung at risk of post-obstructive collapse and infection. Endobronchial resection, dilation and stenting can be performed with either by a rigid or a flexible bronchoscope with good results. Unfortunately, such patients are often referred relatively late in their disease pathway, so while symptom control can be achieved survival is often poor following such procedures.

An occasional complication is the development of a tracheo-oesophageal fistula. This can be very distressing for the patient and is difficult to treat. Stenting can help, but conventional stents have problems, particularly migration. New tracheal Y stents are available that are mostly covered except that part by the right upper lobe, which allows its continued ventilation. Figure 5.8 is a chest radiograph showing a Y-stent in the trachea opening into both main bronchi.

Carcinoid tumours and neuroendocrine cancer

Neuroendocrine cancer is classified into typical carcinoid, atypical carcinoid, large cell neuroendocrine cancer, and small-cell cancer. The last of these is discussed below. Large cell neuroendocrine cancer generally has a poor prognosis but is staged and surgically managed along the same lines as other NSCLC. Atypical carcinoid is usually surgically managed in a similar fashion to NSCLC since nodal spread and distant metastases are fairly common.

In contrast, typical carcinoid has a low rate of nodal spread and distant metastases are rare. In this particular group, providing local resection is complete, lung-preserving strategies are acceptable (Coonar 2005); hence sleeve resections and sublobar resections are more commonly performed. As late recurrence is well recognised, long term follow-up is important.

Surgery for small-cell lung cancer

Most MDTs have considered small-cell lung cancer as a disease in which surgery has a very limited role. However, there are case series of resected small-cell cancer with satisfactory medium- and long-term survival. This must imply that there is a subset of such patients who may benefit from surgery, most probably in the context of multimodality treatment. Currently some MDTs offer surgery to patients staged as having early lung cancer (usually only T1 N0 M0), in combination with chemotherapy, radiotherapy and cranial irradiation (Simon and Turrisi 2007). Less controversial indications for surgery in patients with small-cell lung cancer are surgically resectable recurrent local disease after first-line treatment, the treatment of complications such as a bleeding tumour, and mixed tumours in which the non-small-cell component may not be as well treated by chemoradiotherapy. It is difficult to identify which patients may benefit from surgery as part of first-line treatment is difficult. However, there are proposals for multicentre trials to address this.

Bronchoalveolar cell cancer

This increasingly recognised entity is characterised by a field change that can affect both lungs. The implication of this is that conventional resection may not achieve an adequate margin or local control. A small number of people have been successfully treated by double lung transplantation; however, this is rarely suitable, either because of a shortage of donors or because of contraindications in the recipients. The management overall remains somewhat controversial. An argument can be made for sublobar resections for small lesions with surveillance and consideration of re-resection. Larger tumours with features of invasive adenocarcinoma are generally treated by lobectomy or in some cases pneumonectomy providing the other lung is in good condition.

Postoperative complications, rehabilitation follow-up

Thoracic surgery and general anaesthesia carry the predictable morbidity and other risks common to all types of surgery, which include among other problems pain, bleeding, infection, deep venous thrombosis (DVT), pulmonary embolus (PE), risks to other organs and risk to life. Other risks that are more associated with different types of thoracic surgery include persistent air leaks, bronchopleural fistula and post-peumonectomy problems. Follow-up is important; as with all cancers, recurrence may occur.

Pain

All incisions from a full thoracotomy to single-port mini-VAT procedure can be painful. Strategies to control this are patient-related, anaesthetic and surgical. Good explanation may help the patient to feel in control and this is associated with improved pain control. Pre-incision anaesthesia, perioperative analgesia and appropriate postoperative control have all been shown to be effective. Surgical technique probably has a role to play but is extremely difficult to quantify or to identify specific risk factors. Some authors propose the systematic mobilisation of an intercostal muscle and its associated neurovascular bundle to prevent compression by rib retractors (Cerfolio 2008) The benefits of good early pain control are that it helps coughing and early mobilisation. Failure to achieve this predisposes to retained secretions, chest infection and respiratory failure.

Popular methods of postoperative pain control after thoracotomy include patient-controlled analgesia, extrapleural catheterization to provide regional analgesia, or an epidural, of which there is wider experience. There is increasing evidence that in terms of pain relief they are similar, but an extrapleural catheter is associated with fewer complications.

Bronchopleural fistula and empyema

Complications specific to thoracic surgery include bronchopleural fistula (BPF). This may occur early or late. The immediate management of a large BPF is to protect the remaining lung by positioning the patient on the side with the fistula to prevent fluid contaminating the contralateral lung while surgical advice is sought. The space is usually drained and then the patient is assessed for corrective surgery. Presentations include an increase in expectoration, signs of fever or an abnormal chest radiograph.

Empyema may further complicate this difficult-to-manage complication. An extreme presentation can be an empyema necessitans when the inflected contents of the chest fistulate through the chest wall. Management depends on the condition of the patient and would usually involve prompt drainage, consideration of closure of the fistula and a strategy to sterilise or obliterate the potential space to prevent further empyema.

Post-pneumonectomy pulmonary oedema

Pulmonary oedema after lung resection is an uncommon complication that is particularly recognised after pneumonectomy in the syndrome of so-called 'post-pneumonectomy pulmonary oedema'. The pathophysiology of this is controversial. It may include relatively abrupt increases in blood flow to the remaining lung, but may also be due to aspiration, infection or activation of the systemic inflammatory response from another cause.

Specific complications after pneumonectomy include so-called post-pneumonectomy syndrome, which can be due to mediastinal shift, Post-pneumonectomy syndrome is an uncommon complication and may present with persistent cough and stridor. Surgical correction is possible and there are various techniques to achieve medialisation of the thoracic contents.

Nerve injury

In addition to the intercostal nerves, the intrathoracic nerves that are at risk during surgery are the recurrent laryngeal, vagus and phrenic nerves. The first manifests as a vocal cord injury and is almost always a left-sided injury that occurs in association with either a left upper lobectomy or a left pneumonectomy. It is during dissection of lymph node stations 5 and 6 or the proximal left main pulmonary artery that this is most likely to occur. In the early postoperative period the problem may not declare itself, which can be a consequence of cord oedema secondary to the intubation. After 2–3 days as this fades away, the problem may declare itself in the form of voice change or aspiration. Some may recover over weeks to months. In others, medialisation of the affected cord can be offered by various methods, often with very good results.

Lymph node dissection often effects the vagus. Intraoperatively this can manifest as bradycardia or hypotension. Usually there are no significant lasting effects.

The phrenic nerve is uncommonly injured in the course of the dissection. This can lead to a significant problem due to diaphragm dysfunction. If recovery does not take place within a reasonable time frame – and this can be over months – plication of the hemidiaphragm can be performed either as a VAT or an open procedure. This can produce good outcomes.

Chest drains

Following a thoracotomy or VATS procedure, generally either one or two chest drains are placed in the thoracic cavity. They are connected to an underwater seal and drain air and fluid from the chest. Drains are commonly placed on suction in the immediate post operative period; while the number of drains and use of suction vary between centres, the principle is to remove them once any air-leak has settled and the volume of fluid drained in is acceptably low.

Breathlessness

Some patients experience breathlessness after lung surgery. This may be due to a combination of physical and psychological factors. Physical causes can be due to causes such as reduced lung parenchyma, or factors that lead to increased ventilation/perfusion mismatch (for example, pneumonia or atelectasis). Psychological issues around resection can trigger feelings of dyspnoea even if lung function was excellent before surgery. Supportive care and techniques such as relaxation can help, as can pharmacological treatment in the short term. Referral to a physiotherapist, occupational therapist or specialist nurse may be of benefit. Some people may benefit from oxygen therapy or ventilatory support and specialist assessment should take place.

Chylothorax

An uncommon complication, chylothorax is usually due to injury to the thoracic duct. On the right it is usually associated with station 9 or 8 lymph node dissection, and on the left with surgery around the aortic arch. Sometimes it settles with conservative treatment involving an extremely low-fat diet, but it usually requires surgical closure.

The multidisciplinary team in postsurgical care

Once the patient has had his or her surgery, the prompt availability of results and agreement within the MDT on the next stage of the patient's treatment is valuable. This reduces uncertainty for patients and facilitates their pathway. In our unit, patients are seen as in-patients by specialist cancer nurses within 1–2 days of their surgery for supportive visits and again before discharge when their results may be discussed. If results are not available at the time of discharge, these are communicated to them by telephone or, if more appropriate, in a face-to-face meeting. Patients are usually seen within 2–3 weeks of their surgery by their referring chest physician or oncologist to plan the next step and at around 6–8 weeks for review by the surgical team to deal with any complications, titrate medications (particularly analgesia) and ensure that rehabilitation takes place in a timely fashion. The schematic postoperative treatment is shown in Box 5.7.

Box 5.7   Schematic of postoperative treatment plan

- Surgery.
- Daily review by surgical team.
- Inpatient reviews by a lung cancer specialist nursing team.
- Discharge with communication to family practitioner, referring consultant and if needed community nurses.
- Surgical findings and pathology results discussed at MDT meeting at 1–2 weeks post-op.
- Review by physician or oncologist team at about 2–3 weeks. Further discussion of results; alert surgeon to complications.
- Review by surgical team at about 6 weeks; additional appointments as needed.
- Commence adjuvant treatment as needed.
- Postoperative surveillance programme

Summary

Surgery remains the gold standard for the treatment of non-small-cell lung cancer and is also a valuable method of diagnosis and palliation. Patients undergoing surgical resection of NSCLC must be carefully staged and assessed as thoracic surgery, like any other treatment, carries a degree of risk. In order to increase resection rates, it is important that as many patients as possible are given the opportunity to meet a surgeon.

References

Ali, A., Saee, A., Shamma, L., Rogan, L., Wells, F.C. and Coonar, A.S. (2011) Can mortality after thoracic surgery be prevented? A 5-year institutional review. Oral presentation, SCTS annual meeting, 22 March, 2011.

Berrisford, R., Brunelli, A., Rocco, G., Treasure, T., Utley, M., on behalf of the Audit and guidelines committee of the European Society of Thoracic Surgeons and the European Association of Cardiothoracic Surgeons (2005) The European Thoracic Surgery Database project: modelling the risk of in-hospital death following lung resection. *European Journal of Cardiothoracic Surgery*, **28**, 306-311.

British Thoracic Society (2001) Guidelines on the selection of patients with lung cancer for surgery. *Thorax*, **56** (2), 89-108.

Brunelli, A. (guest ed.) (2008) *Preoperative Evaluation of Lung Resection Candidates*; an issue of *Thoracic Surgery Clinics*. Saunders, Philadelphia.

Brunelli, A., Varela, G., Van Schil, P., *et al.* on behalf of the ESTS Audit and Clinical Excellence Committee (2008) Multicentric analysis of performance after major lung resections by using the European Society Objective Score (ESOS). *European Journal of Cardiothoracic Surgery*, **33**, 284-288.

Brunelli, A., Charloux, A., Bolliger, C.T., *et al.* (2009) The European Respiratory Society and European Society of Thoracic Surgeons clinical guidelines for evaluating fitness for radical treatment (surgery and chemoradiotherapy) in patients with lung cancer. Eur *European Journal of Cardiothoracic Surgery*, **36**, 181-184.

Boushy, S.F., Billig, D.M., North, L.B., *et al.* (1971) Clinical course related to preoperative and postoperative pulmonary function in patients with bronchogenic carcinoma. *Chest*, **59**, 383-391.

Cerfolio, R.J.A., Bryant, S., Patel, B. and Bartolucci, A.A. (2005) Intercostal muscle flap reduces the pain of thoracotomy: a prospective randomized trial. *Journal of Thoracic and Cardiovascular Surgery*, **130**, 987-993.

Cerfolio, R.J., Bryant, A.S. and Maniscalco, L.M. (2008) A nondivided intercostal muscle flap further reduces pain of thoracotomy: a prospective randomized trial. *Annals of Thoracic Surgery*, **85** (6), 1901-1906.

Chamogeorgakis, T., Ieromonachos, C., Georgiannakis, E. and Mallios, D. (2009) Does lobectomy achieve better survival and recurrence rates than limited pulmonary resection for T1N0M0 non-small-cell lung cancer patients? *Interactive Cardiovascular and Thoracic Surgery*, **8** (3), 364-372.

Colice, G.L., Shafazand, S., Griffin, J.P., Keenan, R. and Bolliger, C.T.; American College of Chest Physicians (2007) Physiologic evaluation of the patient with lung cancer being considered for resectional surgery: ACCP evidenced-based clinical practice guidelines (2nd edition). *Chest*, **132** (3 Suppl.), 161S-77S.

Coonar A.S. (2005) Bronchopulmonary carcinoid tumours. In: *The Evidence for Cardiothoracic Surgery* (ed. T. Treasure). TFM Publishing, Lancaster.

Coonar, A.S., Hughes, J., Walker, S., *et al.* (2009a) Implementation of real-time ultrasound in a thoracic surgery practice. *Annals of Thoracic Surgery*, **87** (5), 1577-1581.

Coonar, A.S., Qureshi, N., Smith, I., Wells, F.C., Reisberg, E. and Wihlm, J.M. (2009b) A novel titanium rib bridge system for chest wall reconstruction. *Annals of Thoracic Surgery*, **87** (5), e46-48.

Coonar, A.S., Wihlm, J.M., Wells, F.C. and Qureshi, N. (2011) Intermediate outcome and dynamic computerised tomography after chest wall reconstruction with the STRATOS titanium rib bridge system: video demonstration of preserved bucket-handle rib motion. *Interactive Cardiovascular and Thoracic Surgery*, **12** (1), 80-81.

De Perrot, M., Chernenko, S., Waddell, T.K., *et al.* (2004) Role of lung transplantation in the treatment of bronchogenic carcinomas for patients with end-stage pulmonary disease. *Journal of Clinical Oncology*, **22** (21), 4351-4356.

Fadel, E., Missenard, G., Chapelier, A., *et al.* (2002) En bloc resection of non-small-cell lung cancer invading the thoracic inlet and intervertebral foramina. *Journal of Thoracic and Cardiovascular Surgery*, **123** (4), 676-685.

Falcoz, P.E., Conti, M., Brouchet, L., *et al.* (2007) The Thoracic Surgery Scoring System (Thoracoscore): risk model for in-hospital death in 15,183 patients requiring thoracic surgery. *Journal of Thoracic and Cardiovascular Surgery*, **133**, 325-332.

Ferguson, M.K., Siddique, J. and Karrison, T. (2008) Modeling major lung resection outcomes using classification trees and multiple imputation techniques *European Journal of Cardiothoracic Surgery*, **34**, 1085-1089.

Fischer, S., Darling, G., Pierre, A.F., *et al.* (2008) Induction chemoradiation therapy followed by surgical resection for non-small-cell lung cancer (NSCLC) invading the thoracic inlet. *European Journal of Cardiothoracic Surgery*, **33** (6), 1129-1134.

Flannery, T.W., Suntharalingam, M., Regine, W.F., *et al.* (2005) Long-term survival in patients with synchronous, solitary brain metastasis from non-small-cell lung cancer treated with radiosurgery. *International Journal of Radiation Oncology, Biology, Physics*, **72** (1), 19-23.

Groome, P.A., Bolejack, V., Crowley, J.J., *et al.*; IASLC International Staging Committee; Cancer Research and Biostatistics: Observers to the Committee; Participating Institutions. (2007) The IASLC Lung Cancer Staging Project: validation of the proposals for revision of the, T, N, and M descriptors and consequent stage groupings in the forthcoming (seventh) edition of the TNM classification of malignant tumours. *Journal of Thoracic Oncology*, **2** (8), 694-705.

Goldstraw, P., Crowley, J., Chansky, K., *et al.*; International Association for the Study of Lung Cancer International Staging Committee; Participating Institutions (2007) The IASLC Lung Cancer Staging Project: proposals for the revision of the TNM stage groupings in the forthcoming (seventh) edition of the TNM Classification of malignant tumours. *Journal of Thoracic Oncology*, **2** (8), 706-714. Erratum in: *Journal of Thoracic Oncology* 2007 Oct; **2** (10), 985.

Hughes, B. and MacKay, J. (2008) Analgesia for thoracotomy. *Anaesthesia & Intensive Care Medicine*, **9**, 527-529.

Joshi, G.P., Bonnet, F., Shah, R., *et al.* (2008) A systematic review of randomized trials evaluating regional techniques for postthoracotomy analgesia. *Anesthesia and Analgesia*, **107** (3), 1026-1040.

Katz, J., Jackson, M., Kavanagh, B.P. and Sandler, A.N. (1996) Acute pain after thoracic surgery predicts long-term post-thoracotomy pain. *Clinical Journal of Pain*, **12** (1), 50–55.

Lencioni, R., Crocetti, L., Cioni, R., *et al.* (2008) Radiofrequency ablation of pulmonary tumours: a prospective, intention-to-treat, multicentre clinical trial (the RAPTURE study). *Lancet Oncology*, **9** (7), 621–628.

Lim, E., Baldwin, D., Beckles, M., *et al.*; British Thoracic Society; Society for Cardiothoracic Surgery in Great Britain and Ireland (2010) Guidelines on the radical management of patients with lung cancer. *Thorax*, **65** (Suppl. 3), iii, 1–27.

Miller, J.I. (1993) Physiologic evaluation of pulmonary function in the candidate for lung resection. *Interactive Cardiovascular and Thoracic Surgery*, **105**, 347–352.

Mintz, A., Perry, J., Spithoff, K., Chambers, A. and Laperriere, N. (2007) Management of single brain metastasis: a practice guideline. *Current Oncology*, **14** (4), 131–143.

Olsen, G.N., Block, A.J. and Tobias, J.A. (1974) Prediction of postpneumonectomy pulmonary function using quantitative macroaggregate lung scanning. *Chest*, **66**, 13–16.

Pate, P., Tenholder, M.F., Griffin, J.P., *et al.* (1996) Preoperative assessment of the high-risk patient for lung resection. *Annals of Thoracic Surgery*, **61**, 1494–1500.

Pisters, K.M., Evans, W.K., Azzoli, C.G., *et al.*; Cancer Care Ontario; American Society of Clinical Oncology. Cancer Care Ontario and American Society of Clinical Oncology (2007) Adjuvant chemotherapy and adjuvant radiation therapy for stages I-IIIA resectable non small-cell lung cancer guideline. *Journal of Clinical Oncology* **25** (34), 5506–5518.

Postmus, P.E., Brambilla, E., Chansky, K., *et al.* International Association for the Study of Lung Cancer International Staging Committee; Cancer Research and Biostatistics; Observers to the Committee;Participating Institutions (2007) The IASLC Lung Cancer Staging Project: proposals for revision of the M descriptors in the forthcoming (seventh) edition of the TNM classification of lung cancer. *Journal of Thoracic Oncology*, **2** (8), 686–693.

Rami-Porta, R., Ball, D., Crowley, J., *et al.* International Staging Committee; Cancer Research and Biostatistics; Observers to the Committee; Participating Institutions (2007) The IASLC Lung Cancer Staging Project: proposals for the revision of the T descriptors in the forthcoming (seventh) edition of the TNM classification for lung cancer. *Journal of Thoracic Oncology*, **2** (7), 593–602.

Robinson, L.A., Ruckdeschel, J.C., Wagner, H. and Stevens, C.W. (2007) Treatment of non-small-cell lung cancer-stage IIIA* *Chest*, **132**, 243S–265S.

Rusch, V.W., Crowley, J., Giroux, D.J., *et al.*; International Staging Committee; Cancer Research and Biostatistics; Observers to the Committee; Participating Institutions (2007) The IASLC Lung Cancer Staging Project: proposals for the revision of the N descriptors in the forthcoming seventh edition of the TNM classification for lung cancer. *Journal of Thoracic Oncology*, **2** (7), 603–612.

Russell, H.M. and Ferguson, M.K. (2007) Management of unsuspected N2 disease discovered at thoracotomy. In: *Difficult Decisions in Thoracic Surgery. An Evidence Based Approach* (ed. M.K. Ferguson). Springer, New York.

Samson, D.J., Seidenfeld, J., Simon, G.R., *et al.* (2007) Evidence for management of small-cell lung cancer: ACCP evidence-based clinical practice guidelines (2nd edition). *Chest*, **132**, 314S–323.

Rintoul, R.C., Tournoy, K.G., El Daly, H., *et al.* (2009) EBUS-TBNA for the clarification of PET positive intra-thoracic lymph nodes – an international multi-centre experience. *Thoracic Oncology*, **4** (1), 44–48.

SCTS (2008) *First National Thoracic Surgery Activity & Outcomes Report.* Society for Cardiothoracic Surgery in Great Britain & Ireland. Available at http://www.scts.org/documents/PDF/ThoracicSurgeryReport2008.pdf. Accessed May 2010.

Shen, K.R., Meyers, B.F., Larner, J.M. and Jones, D.R. (2007) Special treatment issues in lung cancer. *Chest,* **132**, 290S–305S. doi:10.1378/chest.07-1382.

Simon, G.R. and Turrisi, A. (2007) Management of small-cell lung cancer: ACCP evidence-based clinical practice guidelines (2nd edition). *Chest* **132** (3 Suppl.), 324S-339.

Tanvetyanon, T., Robinson, L.A., Schell, M.J., *et al.* (2008) Outcomes of adrenalectomy for isolated synchronous versus metachronous adrenal metastases in non-small-cell lung cancer: a systematic review and pooled analysis. *Journal of Clinical Oncology,* **26** (7), 1142-1147.

Waddell, T.K. and Shepherd F.A. (2004) Should aggressive surgery ever be part of the management of small-cell lung cancer? *Thoracic Surgery Clinics,* **14** (2), 271-281.

Yasufuku, K., Nakajima, T., Chiyo, M., Sekine, Y., Shibuya, K. and Fujisawa, T. (2007) Endobronchial ultrasonography: current status and future directions. *Journal of Thoracic Oncology,* **2** (10), 970-979.

Wright, C.D., Gaissert, H.A., Grab, J.D., O'Brien, S.M., Peterson, E.D. and Allen, M.S. (2008) Predictors of prolonged length of stay after lobectomy for lung cancer: a Society of Thoracic Surgeons General Thoracic Surgery Database Risk-Adjustment Model. *Annals of Thoracic Surgery,* **85**, 1857-1865.

Chapter 6
The Nursing Care of Patients with Lung Cancer

Sally Moore

Key points

- Patients with lung cancer and their family members come into contact with a variety of health care and social care professionals, including many nurses working in a number of different roles and settings.
- Patients and family members experience a high number and wide range of physical, social and emotional needs throughout the diagnostic, treatment and follow-up pathway, and beyond.
- Rigorous, comprehensive and on-going assessment is key to meeting patients' and family members' needs, and improving their experience of living with the effects of lung cancer and its treatments.

Introduction

Nurses are recognised as being crucial to the delivery of a comprehensive service to those affected by cancer (Department of Health (DH) 2000, 2007a). More than any other group of health care professionals, nurses have close daily contact with users of health care services and, because of the prevalence of lung cancer, very many nurses, in many different health-care settings, will have direct contact with patients and family members affected by the disease. Thus, nurses, and the quality of their nursing care, are likely to impact significantly on patients' and family members' overall experience of the disease.

Recent documents on cancer and lung cancer focus on the importance of specialist multidisciplinary teams in caring for people with cancer (NICE 2005; DH 2007a; NHS 2009). However, many health care professionals who

Lung Cancer: A Multidisciplinary Approach, First Edition. Edited by Alison Leary.
© 2012 Blackwell Publishing Ltd. Published 2012 by Blackwell Publishing Ltd.

come into contact with patients with lung cancer and their family members, including many nurses, may not necessarily consider themselves as specialists in lung cancer. In the UK, care of cancer patients is mainly undertaken by non-cancer-trained professionals (Closs et al. 1997; DH 2000). The Cancer Reform Strategy (DH 2007a) reminds us just how many health care professionals patients may meet during their cancer experience. The document cites the example of 'Jim', a patient with bowel cancer, who was cared for by 111 different professionals over a 26-month period (p. 75). Many of these professionals were non-cancer-trained. Some worked in hospital settings, others were community based. This situation will be very similar for patients with lung cancer and their family members as they are cared for throughout the illness trajectory from pre-diagnosis, through the diagnostic pathway, treatment, follow-up care, end-of-life care, and into death and bereavement care. The responsibility for delivering effective and high-quality lung cancer services is not solely the domain of specialist lung cancer teams, but lies with any health care professional who is likely to meet patients with lung cancer and their family members, in whatever setting they may be in.

The aim of this chapter, therefore, is to highlight the main issues and areas of care that nurses and other professionals working with patients with lung cancer are likely to face. It is hoped this will provide a useful summary for all nurses who may come into contact with patients with lung cancer regardless of their specialist field and clinical setting.

What are the important issues in relation to lung cancer nursing?

To answer this question, it is necessary to have an understanding of two broad areas:

1. The challenges of lung cancer: nurses require knowledge of the types of lung cancer, the disease and treatment trajectories, and the experience of people affected by the disease.
2. The context in which lung cancer care is delivered: The key strategic and policy initiatives that influence the 'what' and the 'how' of lung cancer service delivery.

The preceding chapters of this book provide in-depth information to update professional knowledge regarding the types of lung cancer, the disease and treatment strategies. This chapter will focus on areas of care that are known to be important in lung cancer care and that present significant challenges for patients and family members. But first, a brief overview of the current context of lung cancer services within the UK will be presented, since this is what shapes our health service and how we, as nurses, are able to deliver care.

Context of lung cancer services

Lung cancer services do not operate in isolation. They are part of a much wider service delivering health and social care. Therefore, the wider health agenda is likely to have a significant influence on lung cancer services. If we initially think in general terms about our health care services in the UK, one of the most important aims currently is to provide high-quality care that is patient centred (DH 2008). Never before has the qualitative aspect of care in improving the patient experience been so high on the health care agenda. And never before has what patients have to say in relation to their health care mattered so much to policy-makers (DH 2007b). Knowing what matters to patients enables us to deliver care that is more likely to meet their needs and expectations.

Quantitative and qualitative work by the Department of Health suggests that what matters to patients in terms of service provision and in their own words is to 'get the basics right; fit in with my life; treat me as a person; and work with me as a partner in my health' (DH 2007b):

1. To get the basics right - don't leave it to chance.
   o Ensure staff are competent.
   o Don't lose my notes.
   o Keep the place clean.
2. To fit in with my life - don't force me to fit in with yours.
   o Make the service easy to access.
   o Give me convenient options.
   o Don't waste my time.
3. To treat me as a person - not a symptom.
   o Listen to me and take me seriously.
   o Understand the wider context of my condition.
   o Treat me with respect and dignity.
4. To work with me as a partner in my health - not just a recipient of care.
   o Encourage me to keep control of the process
   o Equip me to look after my own health
   o Give me the support I need

Written down, these demands seem very simple. But the fact that patients are still requesting these things suggests that current care pathways are constructed in a way that is not meeting these fundamental demands (DH 2007b). Therefore, for us as nurses, planning care pathways that aim to fulfil this wish-list seems a good place to start when we think about meeting the needs of any patient group.

Focusing next on cancer services, the Cancer Reform Strategy (DH 2007a) highlights the following priority areas for improving care:

● Preventing cancer
● Diagnosing cancer earlier

- Ensuring better treatment
- Living with and beyond treatment
- Reducing cancer inequalities
- Delivering care in the appropriate setting

This strategy (and a similar strategy exists in Scotland (Scottish Executive 2001)) spans the cancer trajectory from prevention of cancer through the treatment phases, to living with cancer and/or surviving a diagnosis of cancer, and on to end-of-life care. Once again, patient experience is at the heart of ensuring quality cancer services. The strategy challenges health care professionals to review where services need to be established to ensure that patients' needs and wishes are best met. Each of the six priority areas highlighted in the Cancer Reform Strategy (DH 2007a) has implications for nurses working with people with lung cancer (or people who may be at risk of getting lung cancer), regardless of whether they are working within a specialist lung cancer setting or not.

Thinking specifically about lung cancer services in the UK, our recent national strategies have focused on three main areas:

- Ensuring that patients have early access to investigations and services (particularly at diagnosis)
- Ensuring appropriate patient selection for treatments
- Ensuring that supportive and palliative care measures are fully implemented (NICE 2005; SIGN 2005)

In the past within the UK, it was felt that lung cancer care lacked the energy and resource apparent in other areas of care. Attitudes to lung cancer seemed overly pessimistic, even nihilistic, and services were variable, fragmented and often difficult for patients and their family members to access (NHS Executive 1998; Krishnasamy et al. 2001; Moore et al. 2003). In more recent years, extra funding and resource into lung cancer services have begun to make noticeable improvements. However, it is acknowledged that significant improvements need to be made to ensure that services are equitable throughout the UK (NHS 2009).

The challenges of lung cancer

Previous chapters have highlighted the obvious features of lung cancer that impact on patients' and family members' experience; namely the high morbidity and mortality associated with the disease and its treatments. An awareness of these factors, and the significant impact on patients' and family members' physical, emotional and psychological functioning, will allow nurses to better plan models of care that address the needs of patients and family members. Planning care for patients with lung cancer therefore begins with assessment of individuals' needs.

Patient assessment

Rigorous and comprehensive assessment is key to meeting an individual's specific needs. Systematic assessment of symptoms and concerns is associated with reduced symptom distress (Sarna 1998) and is an essential first step in the process of providing patient-centred care (Richardson *et al.* 2007a). Assessment should be a regular and continuous process throughout the patient's illness since problems and their intensity may vary over time (NICE 2004; Richardson *et al.* 2007a). In the context of lung cancer, given its often short disease trajectory and the fact that patients are often highly symptomatic from the time of diagnosis, it is imperative that assessments are undertaken early. However, assessment of people with cancer, and with lung cancer in particular, seems to present a number of challenges for nurses. We know in general that patients want to be asked about their physical, social and emotional needs. However, evidence suggests that professionals are poor at capturing accurately what patients are trying to tell them (Richardson *et al.* 2007a). Moreover, in lung cancer care, despite many patients experiencing a greater number of unmet needs compared with other patients with cancer (Houts *et al.* 1986; Cooley 2000; Li and Girgis 2006), professionals are poor at assessing needs and patients seem reticent in asking professionals for help (Steele and Fitch 2008). In addition, standardised tools for the assessment of needs in patients with cancer, and specifically for lung cancer, are limited and not widely used in practice (Richardson *et al.* 2007a).

Recent national guidance documents - *Improving Supportive and Palliative Care for Adults with Cancer* (NICE 2004) and the *Holistic Common Assessment of Supportive and Palliative Care Needs for Adults with Cancer* (Cancer Action Team (CAT) 2007) - recommend that patient assessment should be a structured, ongoing process throughout the course of a patient's illness undertaken at the following points:

- Around the time of diagnosis
- At commencement of treatment
- On completion of the primary treatment plan
- In each new episode of disease recurrence
- At the point of recognition of incurability
- At the beginning of end of life
- At the point at which dying is diagnosed
- At any other time the patient may request
- At any other time that a professional carer may judge necessary

It is recommended (CAT 2007) that the patient assessment be divided into five 'domains':

- Background information and assessment preferences
- Physical needs
- Social and occupational needs

- Psychological well-being
- Spiritual well-being

Both guidance documents highlight patients' central role in the assessment process in that 'patients are often the most effective assessors of their needs' (NICE 2004, p. 40). It is therefore suggested that assessment of each domain should be 'concerns-led', focusing upon items of particular concern to the patient (CAT 2007, p. 6). Currently, the guidance focuses on assessment of patients' needs rather than the needs of carers/family members, although it is recognized that carers'/family members' needs might be identified during the course of patient assessment and may need further assessment and action (CAT 2007).

Work is currently underway in the UK to develop a paper-based assessment tool or equivalent for recording the Holistic Common Assessment (CAT 2007). This would provide nurses with a comprehensive screening tool that would ensure that patients' supportive care needs are identified. In the meantime, a useful protocol/tool has been developed by the Yorkshire Lung Cancer Network Nurses to assess and manage the common problems associated with lung cancer (White 2006). The protocol/tool can be found at the Yorkshire Cancer Network website: http://www.ycn.nhs.uk/html/downloads/ycn-lung nurses-follow-upprotocol-july2007.pdf.

Common problems associated with lung cancer

The remainder of this chapter will discuss the management of some of the more common problems and symptoms associated with lung cancer. Problems experienced by patients with lung cancer may relate to the disease itself, effects from treatments, and/or the effects of co-existing disease such as chronic obstructive pulmonary disease, cardiac disease and arthritis. Problems and symptoms are commonly multidimensional and multifactorial. They may occur in isolation, but commonly patients experience a multitude of symptoms, often in clusters (Cooley 2000; Gift et al. 2003, 2004; Chan et al. 2005; Fox and Lyon 2006). Symptom clusters refer to concurrent, related symptoms that may have a synergistic or collective effect on patient outcomes. Some symptom clusters may be related to timing of treatment regimens, and may increase and decline in intensity depending on the treatment involved (Gift et al. 2003, 2004). Others may exist solely because of the disease (Carlssen et al. 2005; Corner et al. 2005; Kitely and Fitch 2006; Fox and Lyon 2006).

Often symptoms are dependent on the burden of cancer and the extent of the disease. Some patients with early stage disease may seem relatively asymptomatic compared with patients with more advanced disease who often experience a multitude of symptoms. However, in the study of Corner et al. (2005) even patients with early stage disease recalled having a number of symptoms for many months. In addition, a number of studies suggest that patients with early stage disease who have undergone curative treatment experience significant residual problems in terms of physical functioning and emotional and social well-being (Dales *et al.* 1994; Zieren *et al.* 1996; Nezu *et al.* 1998; Nugent *et al.* 1999; Handy *et al.* 2002; Sarna *et al.* 2002; Myrdal *et al.* 2003; Uchitomi *et al.* 2003).

Symptoms associated with advanced lung cancer often are accompanied by declining physical, social and emotional functioning (Carlssen *et al.* 2005; Corner *et al.* 2005) and impact significantly on quality of life (Cooley 2000). High levels of symptom distress are associated with a poorer survival (Cooley 2000). Several studies suggest that patients with lung cancer experience more symptom distress than patients with other types of cancer and symptoms are frequently uncontrolled (Cooley 2000). Patients with lung cancer describe their most common problems as:

- Pain
- Breathlessness
- Anorexia
- Fatigue
- Cough
- Low mood
- Social disruption

(Hopwood and Stephens 2000; Krishnasamy *et al.* 2001; Kitely and Fitch 2006). Pain, breathlessness and anorexia are ranked by patients as the most common and also the most intense problems.

This chapter will focus on the management of these patient-reported problems in particular. In addition, superior vena cava obstruction and spinal cord compression are included as these can commonly occur in lung cancer, presenting challenges for both patients and the nurses caring for them. Previous chapters have illustrated the benefit of anti-cancer therapies such as chemotherapy, biological therapies and radiotherapy in palliating and reducing some of the symptoms associated with lung cancer. Despite the potential for significant side effects from these anti-cancer therapies, symptoms such as cough, breathlessness, pain and fatigue can all improve if treatment success-fully controls, or partially controls, the disease (NICE 2005). Therefore, if patients are fit enough to receive anti-cancer therapy, this might be an effective palliative strategy.

Pain

Pain is a common problem in lung cancer, occurring in about half of all patients (Potter and Higginson 2004). Pain may be associated with effects from the primary tumour in the chest or from metastases to other sites, for example to bone. More than one site of pain is common, and chest and lumbar spine are the commonest sites (Potter and Higginson 2004). In most cases, pain corresponds to the locality of the tumour or metastatic disease, but it may be neuropathic in about 30% of cases (Potter and Higginson 2004). Levels of pain can be influenced by emotional elements such as anxiety, fear and hopelessness

Table 6.1 The step process to analgesia (based on the WHO pain relief ladder (WHO 1986).

Step One (mild pain)
  Non-opioid, e.g. paracetamol
  +/– Adjuvant, e.g. ibuprofen or diclofenac

Step Two (mild to moderate pain)
  Mild opioid, e.g. codeine
  +/– Non-opioid, e.g. paracetamol
  +/– Adjuvant, e.g. ibuprofen or diclofenac

Step Three (moderate to severe pain)
  Opioid, e.g. morphine or fentanyl
  +/– Non-opioid, e.g. paracetamol
  +/– Adjuvant, e.g. ibuprofen or diclofenac

(Ahles *et al.* 1983). There are many different pain assessment tools used worldwide but no universally accepted one for the assessment of cancer pain. The European Association of Palliative Care recommend that standardised assessment tools should include visual analogue scales (VAS), numerical rating scales (NRS) and verbal rating scales (VRS) (Caraceni *et al.* 2002).

Pharmacology plays a large role in pain management for patients with lung cancer. The goal of treatment is to optimise pain relief while minimising side effects and inconvenience to the patient. Many analgesic drugs are available in a variety of formulations, giving plenty of opportunity to individualise approaches and research is ongoing to discover preparations that have better analgesic properties with fewer side effects. Research is also ongoing to find better ways to control breakthrough or incident pain more effectively. The WHO analgesic ladder (WHO 1986) remains a useful guide for prescribing analgesics for lung cancer. It is a step process (Table 6.1). If pain relief is not achieved on one step, patients should proceed to the next step.

More recently, Lubbe and Ahmedzai (2004) suggested a revised model of cancer pain management – the pyramid model. This model takes into account the multidimensional nature of pain and incorporates a wider range of pain management strategies. It proposes that each of the four faces of a pyramid corresponds to a type of pain management therapy:

● Face 1: Analgesics including opioids, neurotransmitters, muscle relaxants and anti-inflammatory agents
● Face 2: Oncological treatments including chemotherapy, radiation treatment, hormonal treatment and immune modulation
● Face 3: Surgical and other physical interventions including surgical procedures, nerve blocks, electrical or transcutaneous nerve stimulation (TENS), exercise regimens, physiotherapy and occupational therapy
● Face 4: Psychosocial, complementary and nursing approaches including psychotherapy, cognitive behavioural therapy, acupuncture, massage, aromatherapy, relaxation, distraction therapy, hypnotherapy

Useful adjuvant drugs for the types of pain commonly associated with lung cancer include tricyclic antidepressants or antiepileptic drugs (e.g. amitriptyline, gabapentin or carbemazepine) for neuropathic pain and bisphosphonates for bone pain from metastases. It is vital to remember that psychological, social and spiritual concerns can impact negatively on a person's pain and/or response to analgesia. Focusing on pain solely without addressing other problems in patients' emotional and social world may not prove to be an effective strategy.

Since, within the remit of this chapter, it is not possible to list all strategies that are useful in cancer-related pain, nurses can find a useful guide including both pharmacological and non-pharmacological approaches to pain management at either the National Cancer Institute (NCI) website under 'Pain' (NCI 2009) (www. cancer.gov) or by reading the Scottish national guidelines on cancer pain management (SIGN 2008). Patients can be directed to the Cancer Research UK website, which gives information about the types and causes of cancer pain, and management strategies (www.cancerresearchuk.org.uk).

Breathlessness

Between 55% and 87% of patients with lung cancer will experience breathlessness (Hopwood and Stephens 1995). Patients rate it as one of the three most severe symptoms. Breathlessness is an unpleasant or uncomfortable awareness of breathing or need to breathe (Gift 1990). Patients with lung cancer may experience breathlessness for a variety of reasons such the position of the tumour in the airways or lung, an associated pleural effusion, effects of anti-cancer treatment, anaemia or other co-existing illnesses such as cardiac disease or respiratory airways disease.

For patients with a life-threatening disease such as lung cancer, breathlessness is often a frightening and difficult symptom to manage (O'Driscoll et al. 1999). It is also frightening for family members to witness (O'Driscoll et al. 1999). It is therefore important to address not only the physical component of breathlessness but also the emotional distress it causes to both patients and their carers (Corner et al. 1995). Research suggests that by using non-pharmacological techniques such as breathing retraining, relaxation, pacing activities, goal setting and working with the emotional component of breathlessness, in conjunction with pharmacology, nurses can significantly improve the experience of breathlessness for patients with cancer (Bredin et al. 1999). Corner and O'Driscoll (1999) have developed a breathlessness assessment tool for use in the lung cancer setting to assist nurses in their assessment and management of patients. It combines assessment of the physical experience of breathlessness with an exploration of the emotional and social impact also.

Drug therapy for breathlessness includes the use of opioids, benzodiazepines and oxygen. Little evidence exists confirming the effectiveness of these in reducing breathlessness. However, a recent Cochrane review suggests that morphine may decrease the level of distress patients experience from breathlessness (Jennings et al. 2003). Some patients find anxiolytics such as the benzodiazepines (lorazepam and diazepam) helpful in relieving breathlessness because of their sedative effect, which like that of morphine may depress respiration and thus dull the sensation of breathlessness for patients. Anxiolytics may also reduce anxiety related to breathlessness and assist the action of breathing by their muscle relaxation effect.

Although oxygen is widely used by patients with cancer who are breathless, there are no studies confirming its benefit in the absence of hypoxia. People without hypoxia may gain as much benefit from a cool draft of air across the face from a fan (Schwartzstein et al. 1987). Oxygen may have a placebo effect for some patients, but psychological dependence on its use may decrease physical functioning and increase social isolation. To avoid giving oxygen inappropriately, it should be initially administered for a short trial period and only continued if the patient derives clear benefit from it.

Corticosteroids may have a useful effect on breathlessness when there is thought to be oedema around the tumour exacerbating airways obstruction, superior vena cava obstruction, lymphangitis carcinomatosa, radiation-induced pneumonitis, chronic airways disease or asthma.

Poor appetite

Poor appetite is common in patients with lung cancer (Cooley 2000). Weight loss and changes in physique can cause significant emotional distress and concern particularly for family members. Poor appetite and weight loss may be caused by the effects of the cancer itself, by other symptoms such as breathlessness, constipation and pain, by effects from anti-cancer treatment such as chemotherapy and radiotherapy, and by emotional factors. Weight loss is associated with increased mortality and poor prognosis (Brundage et al. 2002).

Some patients with lung cancer will suffer from cancer cachexia syndrome (CCS), which is a syndrome of progressive weight loss, anorexia, and persistent erosion of body cell mass in response to a malignant growth (Bosaeus 2008). It is thought to be caused by complex changes in cytokine and hormone levels. Although CCS is often associated with pre-terminal patients with disseminated disease, it may be present in the early stages of tumour growth before any signs or symptoms of malignancy. Unlike in starvation, the weight loss associated with CCS will continue despite increased energy intake. Therefore, if the underlying cancer remains uncontrolled, strategies aimed at improving appetite and energy intake may prove futile.

As with all symptoms, a thorough assessment of the problem is vital to identify the most helpful strategies. Firstly, it is important where possible to correct any factors that may inhibit oral intake such as dry mouth, mucositis, infection and nausea. Appetite may be stimulated with the use of alcohol before meals or drugs such as megestrol acetate or corticosteroids, although the benefits of these are limited. Nutritional supplements in liquid or powder forms can be given. An early referral to a dietician may be helpful. However, in advanced cancer, it may be important to recognise and acknowledge with the patient and family members that weight gain may not be possible and that the goal should be to maintain weight as far as possible.

The following simple advice may be helpful for patients and family members.

- Keep the mouth as moist and clean as possible.
- Eat small meals and snacks instead of large meals.
- Drink plenty of fluids, particularly nourishing drinks and nutritional supplements.
- Eat what you fancy.
- Choose a wide variety of foods to avoid getting bored with the same flavours.
- Allow others to prepare food for you.
- If you have to attend the hospital regularly, or if you are out, take a snack with you that you enjoy.
- If you have difficulty chewing or swallowing, try a soft or puréed diet.
- Try not to become anxious over not eating.
- If you are a carer, remember that there is a fine balance between encouragement and nagging. Try not to become over-anxious about a loved one's dietary intake.

Fatigue

Fatigue is described by Piper *et al.* (1987) as 'an unremitting and overwhelming lack of energy and an inability to maintain usual routines'. Fatigue is a common symptom of the disease itself, but is often compounded by anti-cancer treatments, other drugs, other existing medical conditions and age. Strategies addressing the cause of fatigue such as correcting anaemia and insomnia and controlling disabling symptoms such as pain and breathlessness are vital first steps. Exploring and advising on the role of nutrition, exercise and the planning of activities to help better manage fatigue may also help patients. Increasingly, evidence is suggesting that physical activity may benefit people with cancer who are experiencing fatigue (Dimeo 2001; Lucktar-Flude *et al.* 2009). Addressing symptoms such as anxiety and depression may help patients feel more energised also. Table 6.2 is a list of strategies that patients may find helpful in managing fatigue.

Cough

Cough can also be a troublesome symptom for people with lung cancer and one that is often difficult to ameliorate. It can be caused by the tumour itself; either its position or its effect (such as pleural effusion or lymphangitis for example), infection, other existing medical conditions and/or anti-cancer therapies such as chemotherapy-induced pulmonary or cardiac toxicity or radiotherapy-induced pneumonitis. The initial focus to relieve cough, as with

Table 6.2 Strategies for patients that may help alleviate fatigue (adapted from Macmillan Cancer Support 2007 guidance).

Exercise	Regular, light exercise may decrease fatigue and improve sleep. Plan some light exercise or activity into the day. Find a balance between activity and rest, and exercise in a way that allows the muscles to recover after activity.
Diet	Try to take advantage of the times when appetite is best. Drink plenty of fluids. Try new foods or eat foods that taste best. Eat little and often.
Sleep	Sleep as much as needed to feel refreshed but not more than necessary, especially during the day as this can make you feel sluggish and disrupt sleep patterns at night. Limiting time in bed seems to produce better quality sleep. Wake up at the same time every day. Reduce noise when sleeping. Avoid stimulants such as coffee prior to sleep. Keep a steady temperature in the room.
Plan activities	Plan activities ahead of time so that there is time for activities and time for rest. Plan your day so that you have time to rest and do the things you want to do most. Spread tasks out over the week. Doing things for yourself is very important, but try not to feel guilty if you have to ask other people to help. Ask others to do heavy work. Sit down to do chores wherever possible.
Relaxation	Make time for relaxation. Avoid stressful situations whenever possible as stress uses up energy. Talk to others about anything that is worrying you. Try distraction techniques such as reading and music to take your mind away from worrying thoughts.

breathlessness, is therapy aimed at addressing the underlying cause in the first instance if at all possible – for example, to drain any pleural effusion present, or insert a stent to open up an obstructed airway.

Management of disease-related cough is guided by whether the cough produces sputum or is non-productive. Adequate hydration, air humidification and chest physiotherapy can help with expectoration of sputum. Nebulised saline may help patients who complain of a dry cough, although there is little evidence to support its use. Some patients may find an expectorant helpful, although evidence to support their use is lacking. A mucolytic such as carbocysteine may reduce sputum viscosity and thereby promote expectoration and reduce cough. Where the aim of treatment is to suppress the cough, trial of an opiate such as pholcodine, codeine or morphine can often prove useful. Methadone linctus may be tried if these fail, but care must be taken as its effects can be cumulative. Corticosteroids may also benefit some patients but the cough often returns once these are withdrawn.

Superior vena cava obstruction

In lung cancer, superior vena cava obstruction (SVCO) is present at diagnosis in 10% of patients with small-cell lung cancer (SCLC) and 1.7% of patients with non-small-cell lung cancer (NSCLC) (Rowell and Gleeson 2001). SVCO can occur when there is occlusion of the superior vena cava causing congestion of the veins draining into the superior vena cava from the head, neck, upper extremities, and upper thorax. Occlusion may be partial or complete as a result of external compression by the tumour or lymph nodes (i.e. occlusion from outside the vein) or internal obstruction by thrombosis or tumour (i.e. arising inside the vein). SVCO can cause a number of symptoms in patients that can vary in speed of onset and severity, and can be life-threatening:

- Breathlessness, worse on lying flat
- Choking sensation
- Headache and/or a feeling of fullness in the head
- Neck and facial swelling
- Early morning oedema of the eyelids making it hard for the patient to open their eyes
- Trunk and arm swelling
- Dilated veins on neck, chest and arms (may cause duskiness of skin in those areas)
- Visual changes
- Dizziness

(Haapoja and Blendowski 1999; Buckley 2008). Patients may notice increased symptoms in the morning after sleeping in a supine position, or with position changes such as bending forward. High-dose steroids, and sometimes diuretics, are used in the short term to relieve symptoms. Thrombolytic therapy may be used if a thrombosis is suspected. However, the risk of haemorrhage with anticoagulant therapy must be weighed against the possible benefits. A Cochrane review of the effectiveness of treatments in the management of SVCO found that morbidity following stent insertion was greater if thrombolytics were administered (Rowell and Gleeson 2001). Treatment options include insertion of stent, chemotherapy, and/or radiotherapy.

The development of SVCO can be a frightening experience for patients and their family members. Nursing interventions include the early recognition of symptoms, provision of information and support to patients and family members to help them manage the effects of symptoms and treatment effects, symptom management, and ensuring ease of access for patients to obtain further advice or review.

Spinal cord compression

Malignant spinal cord compression (SCC) occurs when there is pathological vertebral body collapse or direct tumour growth causing compression of the spinal cord or cauda equina (National Collaborating Centre for Cancer (NCCC) 2008). This can potentially lead to permanent loss of neurological function resulting in paraplegia if the pressure of the tumour on the spinal cord is not relieved quickly (Levack et al. 2002). Early diagnosis and treatment is essential to prevent permanent neurological damage, as once paraplegia develops it is usually irreversible (NCCC 2008). Survival for patients with lung cancer who develop SCC is often extremely poor, although there can be significant variability. One series reports a range of survival from 0 to 132 months (Bach *et al.* 1992). However, usually median survival is between 1 and 2.5 months (Loblaw *et al.* 2003). Patients with cancer who present with widespread malignancy and those with known spinal metastases are at higher risk of SCC (NCCC 2008).

The presenting signs and symptoms depend on the level of the metastatic tumour, the degree of cord compression and the duration of tumour involvement. Symptoms may develop gradually and be sparse, or develop suddenly. Symptoms may include:

- Back pain (may be localized, radiating, or both, and often precedes signs related to cord compression)
- Weakness in one or both limbs
- Changes in sensation including paraesthesia, decreased sensation and numbness in the arms, hands, fingers legs, feet, toes and trunk
- Impotence, bladder and bowel dysfunction (urinary retention, incontinence or constipation)

(Bach *et al.* 1992; NCCC 2008). If SCC is suspected, high-dose steroids and analgesia should be commenced. Magnetic resonance imaging (MRI) is used to diagnose SCC. Treatment of SCC should commence ideally within 24 hours of the confirmed diagnosis (NCCC 2008). Treatment options depend on the fitness and likely prognosis of the patient and include surgery followed by radiotherapy if successful, or radiotherapy alone. Guidelines suggest dexamethasone 16 mg daily in patients awaiting surgery or radiotherapy (unless otherwise contraindicated). After surgery, or the start of radiotherapy, the dose should be reduced gradually over 5-7 days and stopped. If neurological function deteriorates at any time, the dose should be increased temporarily.

Where there is severe mechanical pain suggestive of spinal instability or neurological symptoms, guidelines suggest that patients should lie flat with neutral spine alignment until bony and neurological stability are ensured. If significant increase in pain or neurological symptoms occurs when patients begin gradual sitting and mobilisation, they should return to a position in which the symptoms reverse. In patients who are not fit for surgery or radiotherapy, there should be a full discussion of the risks, and they should be helped to position themselves and mobilize as symptoms permit (NCCC 2008).

Nursing care involves the early recognition of symptoms, and prompt referral for medical review and management. It may also involve ensuring adequate pain management (including the use of bisphosphonates), interventions for thromboprophylaxis if mobility is impaired, management of pressure areas, bladder and bowel continence management, maintaining circulatory and respiratory functioning, and ensuring early referral and access to rehabilitation therapists, for example physiotherapists and occupational therapists.

The psychological and social consequences of SCC can be huge, particularly where functional ability is severely affected. Nurses, with members of the wider multiprofessional team, can help patients and family members with decisions regarding which mode of therapy, if any, is appropriate for them by exploring the patient's goals, the likely outcomes of each therapy (e.g. pain relief or preservation or return of function), the beneficial and adverse effects of therapy, the likely duration of in-patient and rehabilitation stays, and the estimated survival times with and without therapy (NCCC 2008).

Low mood

The psychological morbidity that accompanies a diagnosis of cancer is well documented (Maguire 1985; Holland 1989). Patients with lung cancer have high levels of emotional distress (Houts et al. 1986; Hopwood and Stephens 2000; Zabora et al. 2001; Carlsen et al. 2005) and this interferes with and impacts negatively on their quality of life (Sarna et al. 2005; Fox and Lyon 2006). A variety of factors can negatively impact a person's psychological well-being. These can relate to:

- The patients' disease status; for example, advanced stage of disease, poorly controlled symptoms, threat of death
- The patients' experience of care; for example, difficult diagnostic pathway, poor relationships with health care providers, lack of information
- Social issues; for example, lack of supportive relationships, financial concerns, spiritual concerns
- Psychological factors; for example, history of depression

Patients with lung cancer consider psychosocial concerns as priorities (Sarna et al. 2005; Krishnasamy et al. 2007). However, there is evidence that these needs are often unrecognised and poorly addressed by health care professionals (Houts et al. 1986; Fox and Lyon 2006; Krishnasamy et al. 2007).

National cancer guidance in the UK urges health care professionals to assess patients' and family members' psychological health on a regular basis throughout the patient pathway (NICE 2004). The guidance suggests a four-level model of psychological assessment and support (Table 6.3), wherein all nurses should be competent to undertake an initial psychological assessment and be able to refer patients and family members to more specialist services where appropriate.

Providing care that is supportive and holistic may help prevent low mood and psychological distress. Ensuring that care is coordinated and timely and that patients and family members are kept well-informed, and providing continuity of care may help patients' psychological adjustment to cancer and its treatments (London and South East Lung Cancer Forum for Nurses 2004). Developing therapeutic relationships with patients and their families may improve patients' coping, and enable nurses to

Table 6.3 Recommended model of professional assessment and support.

Level	Group	Assessment	Intervention
1	All health and social care professionals	Recognition of psychological needs	Effective information giving, compassionate communication and general psychological support
2	Health and social care professionals with additional expertise	Screening for psychological distress	Psychological techniques such as problem solving
3	Trained and accredited professionals	Assessed for psychological distress and diagnosis of some psychopathology	Counselling and specific psychological interventions such as anxiety management and solution-focused therapy, delivered according to an explicit theoretical framework
4	Mental health specialists	Diagnosis of psychopathology	Specialist psychological and psychiatric interventions such as psychotherapy, including cognitive behavioural therapy (CBT)

recognise low mood, anxiety and depression early and offer treatment strategies or referrals to specialists appropriately.

Social disruption

A diagnosis of lung cancer significantly impacts social functioning; enforcing alterations in work, family roles and social activities for both patients and family members (Ryan 1996; Ramalingham and Balani 2002). Social changes may cause financial difficulties if employment and earnings are lost or reduced, and increases in living costs because of demands of the illness and treatment schedule. Accommodation may become unsuitable if there are functional limitations.

The profound impact of a cancer diagnosis on the family and friends of cancer patients is increasingly recognised also (Hinds 1985; Higginson *et al.* 1990; Glajchen 2004; Osse *et al.* 2006; Macmillan Cancer Support 2006). Family members experience a range of emotional disturbance as well as financial and practical concerns (Harrison *et al.* 1995; Payne *et al.* 1999; Plant 2000). Cancer may put intolerable strain on family daily routines, communication and relationships (Lewis 1993; Macmillan Cancer Support 2006). Spouses of patients with lung cancer report not sharing their fears with the patient, changes in the degree of closeness of the relationship, and increased stress and feeling alone (Cooper 1984). For close family and friends, providing support and care for the patient can be immensely rewarding, but it can also be burdensome and stressful (Plant 2000; Haley *et al.* 2001; Thomas *et al.* 2002).

Despite this growing awareness in the cancer literature, assessment and support of family members' needs is not given high priority within everyday clinical practice (Moore *et al.* 2006a; Osse *et al.* 2006). This may be due to health professionals' lack of time and resource, or a concern they will not have the knowledge and skills to be able to respond adequately to the family members' needs for support (Osse *et al.* 2006). Health care professionals may assume family members' willingness to undertake a care-giving role without asking, and family members are often reticent in voicing their own needs or concerns (Plant 2000; Thomas *et al.* 2002; Isaksen *et al.* 2003; Glajchen 2004). Moreover, family members take on the role of caregiver with little preparation and guidance; often in sudden and extreme circumstances, and it is only when things go wrong that the importance of the informal care-giving role is recognised and services are forced to respond (James 1989; Harding and Higginson 2003).

It is important that this broader social impact of lung cancer is recognised and addressed by health care professionals. Nurses are in an ideal position to make an initial social-needs assessment and refer to the relevant specialists and outside agencies where necessary. Assessment should be ongoing and undertaken with both the patient and family to ensure that all needs are considered. There are many professionals and outside agencies that can have a significant role in helping patients with lung cancer to maximise their social functioning, including:

- Occupational therapists
- Physiotherapists
- Palliative care teams
- Social services
- Benefits advisors
- Housing teams
- General practitioners
- Chaplains
- District nursing teams

A recent pilot project suggests that proactive support by nurses can lead to benefits for family members of people with lung cancer (Plant *et al.* 2006). Key components of this intervention that family members identified as supportive included being listened to by someone who could facilitate emotional expression, being provided with individually tailored information, and receiving practical help and advice (Richardson *et al.* 2007b).

In summary, nurses can make a significant difference in the way that patients with lung cancer and their family members experience the impact of lung cancer. Strategies initiated by nurses can lead to improvements in how well patients and their families manage, and cope with, the physical, psychological and social effects of this disease. Comprehensive and ongoing assessment of need at key points through the disease and treatment pathway is essential.

The role of the specialist nurse

Specialist nurses play a significant role in the management of patients with cancer (National Cancer Action Team 2010). In lung cancer, research suggests the involvement of specialist nurses can lead to positive outcomes and improve the experience of care.

Titles are varied, ranging through respiratory nurse specialists, thoracic nurse specialists, lung cancer nurse specialists and palliative care nurse specialists (Moore 2002). Some specialist nurses care for patients at specific time points in the disease or treatment trajectory, for example during the diagnostic pathway prior to referral to oncology teams, during oncological management, or during the palliative phase of the illness. Alternatively, some nurse specialist roles may span the whole patient journey. Whatever the setting, the role focuses on the supportive care of patients and their family members, as well as having an education and research component. Nurse specialists aim to ensure that care incorporates not only the physical aspect of disease management but also the emotional and social needs of patients and their family members. They are able to work with other colleagues to help bridge the gaps between the various professionals and services involved to ensure a more coherent and streamline service for patients (London and South East Lung Cancer Forum for Nurses 2004).

Specific areas of care identified as integral to the role of the nurse specialist in lung cancer care include:

- Development of a therapeutic relationship over time with individual patients and their carers based on sensitivity, responsiveness and honesty
- Giving, clarifying and reinforcing information over time about:
  - The disease and likely disease process
  - Diagnostic investigations
  - The aims, likely effects and possible side effects of treatment
  - Possible future outcomes
  - Supportive services available
- Acting as a key resource for patients so that they have access to prompt and expert help and advice. Ensuring that patients are aware of how to access help at times of emergency or outside normal working hours
- Accurate and ongoing assessment of physical, psychological and social needs and development of appropriate management strategies to meet such needs
- Liaison with, and early referral to, other specialist teams or agencies who may be better placed to meet such needs
- Active participation within the Lung Cancer Team to ensure that care is streamlined and coordinated and that delays are kept to a minimum
- Rapid communication and liaison with primary and secondary care teams, and between hospital teams and departments
- Strategic planning for future care needs of patients

- Close liaison with, and early referral to, specialist palliative care services, where appropriate, to ensure smooth and timely transition from acute to palliative services

In England and Wales, there are just under 250 site-specific lung cancer nurse specialists (Trevatt and Leary 2009). Given that the number of newly diagnosed patients with lung cancer each year is approximately 39 000 (CRUK 2009), individual nurse specialist case-loads are high. In practice this means that nurse specialists may risk 'spreading themselves thinly' and thereby run the risk of diluting their beneficial effect (Richardson *et al.* 2002; Moore *et al.* 2006b). It is imperative therefore that all nurses caring for patients with lung cancer understand the far-reaching implications of this disease and work proactively to address patients' problems and concerns.

Summary

Lung cancer significantly impacts on all aspects of patients' and their family members' physical, social and emotional lives. Nurses are in an ideal position to assess and intervene to help patients manage the effects of the disease and treatments, and thereby live better with the disease. In a disease such as lung cancer where the morbidity and mortality are so high, supportive and palliative care is paramount to ensure that patients and their family member achieve the maximum quality of life possible. Much can be gained by effective and timely collaboration with colleagues from the multiprofessional team to optimise management and support.

References

Ahles, T.A., Blanchard, E.B. and Ruckdeschel, J.C. (1983) The multidimensional nature of cancer related pain. *Pain*, **17**, 277–288.

Bach, F., Agerlin, N., Sorensen, J.B., *et al.* (1992) Metastatic spinal cord compression secondary to lung cancer. *Journal of Clinical Oncology*, **10** (11), 1781–1787.

Bosaeus, I. (2008) Nutritional support in multimodal therapy for cancer cachexia. *Supportive Care in Cancer*, **16** (5), 447–451.

Bredin, M., Corner, J., Krishnasamy, M., Plant, H., Bailey, C. and A'Hern, R. (1999) Multicentre randomised controlled trial of nursing intervention for breathlessness in patients with lung cancer. *British Medical Journal*, **318**, 901–904.

Brundage, M.D., Davies, D. and Mackillop, W.J. (2002) Prognostic factors in non-small-cell lung cancer. A decade of progress. *Chest*, **122** (3), 1037–1057.

Buckley, J. (2008) *Palliative Care: An Integrated Approach*. Wiley and Sons Ltd, Chichester.

Caraceni, A., Chemy, N., Fainsinger, R., Kaasa, S., Poulain, P. and Radbruch, L. (2002) Pain measurement tools and methods in clinical research in palliative care: recommendations of an expert working group of the European Association of Palliative Care. *Journal of Pain and Symptom Management*, **23** (3), 239–255.

Cancer Action Team (2007) *Holistic Common Assessment of Supportive and Palliative Care Needs for Adults with Cancer: Assessment Guidance*. National Cancer Action Team, London.

Carlsen, K., Jensen, A. and Jacobsen, E. (2005) Psychosocial aspects of lung cancer. *Lung Cancer*, **47**, 293–300.

Chan, C.W., Richardson, A. and Richardson, J. (2005) A study to assess the existence of the symptom cluster of breathlessness, fatigue and anxiety in patients with advanced lung cancer. *European Journal of Oncology Nursing*, **9**, 325–333.

Closs, S.J., Ferguson, A. and Rae, M.J. (1997) Developing local cancer nursing services in the wake of a national policy. *Journal of Cancer Nursing*, **1** (1), 1624.

Cooley, M.E. (2000) Symptoms in adults with lung cancer. A systematic research review. *Journal of Pain and Symptom Management*, **19**, 137–153.

Cooper, E.T. (1984) A pilot study on the effects of the diagnosis of lung cancer on family relationships. *Cancer Nursing*, **7** (4), 301–308.

Corner, J., Hopkinson, J., Fitzsimmons, D., Barclay, S., Muers, M. (2005) Is late diagnosis of lung cancer inevitable? Interview study of patients' recollections of symptoms before diagnosis. *Thorax*, **60**, 314–331.

Corner, J. and O'Driscoll, M. (1999) Development of a breathlessness assessment guide for use in palliative care. *Palliative Medicine*, **13**, 375–384.

Corner, J., Plant, H. and Warner, L. (1995) Developing a nursing approach to managing dyspnoea in lung cancer. *International Journal of Palliative Nursing*, **1**, 5–10.

Dales, R.E., Belanger, R., Shamji, F.M. Leech, J., Crepeau, A. and Sachs, H.J. (1994) Quality of life following thoracotomy for lung cancer. *Journal of Clinical Epidemiology*, **47**, 1443–1449.

DH (2000) *The Nursing Contribution to Cancer Care. A Strategic Programme of Action in Support of the National Cancer Programme*. Department of Health, London.

DH (2007a) *Cancer Reform Strategy*. Department of Health, London.

DH (2007b) *What Matters to Our Patients, Public and Staff*. Department of Health, London.

DH (2008) *High Quality Care for All. NHS Next Stage Review Final Report*. Department of Health, London.

Dimeo, F.C. (2001) Effects of exercise on cancer-related fatigue. *Cancer*, **92** (6, Suppl.), 1689–1693.

Fox, S.W. and Lyon, D.E. (2006) Symptom clusters and quality of life in survivors of lung cancer. *Oncology Nursing Forum*, **33** (5), 931–936.

Gift, A. (1990) Dyspnea. *Nursing Clinics of North America*, **25** (4), 955–965.

Gift, A.G., Stommel, M., Jablonski, A. and Given, W. (2003) A cluster of symptoms over time in patients with lung cancer. *Nursing Research*, **52**, 393–400.

Gift, A.G., Jablonski, A. and Stommel, M. (2004) Symptom clusters in elderly patients with lung cancer. *Oncology Nursing Forum*, **31**, 202–212.

Glajchen, M. (2004) The emerging role and needs of family caregivers in cancer care. *Journal of Supportive Oncology*, **2** (2), 145–155.

Haapoja, I. and Blendowski, C. (1999) Superior vena cava syndrome. *Seminars in Oncology Nursing*, **15**, 183–189.

Haley, W., LaMonde, L., Han, B., Narramore, S. and Schonwetter, R. (2001) Family caregiving in hospice: effects on psychological and health functioning among spousal caregivers of hospice patients with lung cancer or dementia. *Hospice Journal*, **15** (4), 1–18.

Handy, J.R., Asaph, J.W., Skokan, L., *et al.* (2002) What happens to patients undergoing lung cancer surgery? Outcomes and quality of life before and after surgery. *Chest*, **122** (1), 21–30.

Harding, R. and Higginson, I. (2003) What is the best way to help caregivers in cancer and palliative care? A systematic literature review of interventions and their effectiveness. *Palliative Medicine*, **17**, 63-74.

Harrison, J., Haddad, P. and Maguire, P. (1995) The impact of cancer on key relatives: a comparison of relative and patient concerns. *European Journal of Cancer*, **31A** (11), 1736-1740.

Hinds, C. (1985) The needs of families who care for patients with cancer at home: are we meeting them? *Journal of Advanced Nursing*, **10** (6), 575-581.

Higginson, I., Wade, A. and McCarthy, M. (1990) Palliative care: views of patients and their families. *British Medical Journal*, **301**, 277-281.

Holland, J.C. (1989) *Lung Cancer*. In: *Handbook of Psychoonocology* (eds J.C. Holland and Rowland, J.H), p. 184. Oxford University Press, New York.

Hopwood, P. and Stephens, R.J. (1995) Symptoms at presentation for treatment in patients with lung cancer: implications for the evaluation of palliative treatment. The Medical Research Council (MRC) Lung Cancer Working Party. *British Journal of Cancer*, **71**, 633-636.

Hopwood, P. and Stephens, R. (2000) Depression in patients with lung cancer: prevalence and risk factors derived from quality of life data. *Journal of Clinical Oncology*, **18** (4), 893-903.

Houts, P.A., Yasko, J.M., Kahn, B., *et al*. (1986) Unmet psychological, social, and economic needs of persons with cancer in Pensylvania. *Cancer*, **58**, 2355-2361.

Isaksen, A.S., Thuen, F. and Hanestad, B. (2003) Patients with cancer and their close relatives: experiences with treatment, care and support. *Cancer Nursing*, **26** (1), 68-74.

James, N. (1989) Emotional labour: skill and work in the social regulation of feelings. *Sociological Review*, **37** (1), 15-42.

Jennings, A.L., Davies, A.N., Higgins, J.P.T. and Broadley, K. (2003) *Opioids for the Palliation of Breathlessness in Terminal Illness (Cochrane Review)*. In: The Cochrane Library 2003. Issue 3. Update Software, Oxford.

Kitely, C.A. and Fitch, M.I. (2006) Understanding the symptoms experienced by individuals with lung cancer. *Canadian Oncology Nursing Journal*, **16** (1), 25-30.

Krishnasamy, M., Wells, M. and Wilkie, E. (2007) Patients and carer experiences of care provision after a diagnosis of lung cancer in Scotland. *Supportive Care Cancer*, **15**, 327-332.

Krishnasamy, M., Wilkie, E. and Haviland, J. (2001) Lung cancer health care needs assessment: Patients' and informal carers' response to a national mail questionnaire survey. *Palliative Medicine*, **15**, 213-227.

Levack, P., Graham, J. and Collie, D. (2002) Don't wait for a sensory level-listen to the symptoms: a prospective audit of the delays in diagnosis of malignant cord compression. *Clinical Oncology*, **14**, 472-480.

Lewis, F.M. (1993) Psychological transitions and the family's work in adjusting to cancer. *Seminars in Oncology Nursing*, **9** (2), 127-129.

Li, J. and Girgis, A. (2006) Supportive care needs: Are patients with lung cancer a neglected population? *Psycho-oncology*, **15**, 509-516.

Loblaw, D.A., Laperriere, N.J. and Mackillop, W.J. (2003) A population-based study of malignant spinal cord compression in Ontario. *Clinical Oncology (Royal College of Radiologists)*, **15** (4), 211-217.

London and South East Lung Cancer Forum for Nurses (2004) Guidelines on the role of the nurse specialist in supporting patients with lung cancer. *European Journal of Cancer Care*, **13**, 344-348.

Lubbe, S. and Ahmedzai, S. (2004) A new approach for cancer pain management – the pyramid model. *Progress in Palliative Care*, **12** (6), 287-292.

Luctkar-Flude, M., Groll, D., Woodend, K. and Tranmer, J. (2009) Fatigue and physical activity in older patients with cancer: a six-month follow-up study. *Oncology Nursing Forum*, **36** (2), 194-202.

Macmillan Cancer Support (2007) *Coping with Fatigue*. Available at http://www.macmillan.org.uk/Cancerinformation/Livingwithandaftercancer/Symptomssideeffects/Fatigue/Fatiguecancer.aspx. Accessed 19 October 2009.

Macmillan Cancer Support (MCS) (2006) *Worried Sick: The Emotional Impact of Cancer*. MCS, London. Available at http://www.macmillan.org.uk/Documents/Support_Material/Get_involved/Campaigns/Impact_of_cancer_english.pdf. Accessed 20 October 2009.

Maguire, P. (1985) The psychological impact of cancer. *British Journal of Hospital Medicine*, **34** (2), 100-103.

Moore, S., Corner, J., Haviland, J., *et al.* (2002a) Nurse led follow up and conventional medical follow up in the management of lung cancer: randomised trial. *British Medical Journal*, **325**, 1145-1147.

Moore, S. (2002b) A survey of nurse specialists working with patients with lung cancer. *European Journal of Oncology Nursing*, **6** (3), 169-175.

Moore, S., Halliday, D. and Plant, H. (2003) Evidence based service for patients with lung cancer. *Cancer Nursing Practice*, **2** (2), 35-39.

Moore, S., Sherwin, A., Medina, J., Ream, E., Plant, H. and Richardson, A. (2006a) A prospective audit of nurse specialist contact with families and carers of patients with lung cancer. *European Journal of Oncology Nursing*, **10** (3), 207-211.

Moore, S., Wells, M., Plant, H., Corner, J., Fuller, F. and Wright, M. (2006b) Nurse Specialist led follow-up in lung cancer. The experience of developing and delivering a new model of care. *European Journal of Oncology Nursing*, **10**, 364-337.

Myrdal, G., Vlatysdottir, S., Lambe, M. and Stahle, E. (2003) Quality of life following lung cancer surgery. *Thorax*, **58** (3), 194-197.

National Cancer Action Team (2010) *Excellence in Cancer Care: The Contribution of the Clinical Nurse Specialist*. Avaialble at: http://www.macmillan.org.uk/Documents/AboutUs/Commissioners/ExcellenceinCancerCaretheContributionoftheClinicalNurseSpecialist.pdf. Accessed 11 July 2011).

National Cancer Institute (NCI) (2009) *Pain*. Available at http://www.cancer.gov/cancertopics/pdq/supportivecare/pain/Patient/page1. Accessed 19 October 2009.

National Collaborating Centre for Cancer (NCCC) (2008) *Metastatic Spinal Cord Compression: Diagnosis and Management of Patients at Risk of or with Metastatic Spinal Cord Compression*. NCCC, Cardiff.

National Institute for Health and Clinical Excellence (NICE) (2004) *Guidance on Cancer Services. Improving Supportive and Palliative Care for Adults with Cancer. The Manual*. NICE, London.

National Institute for Health and Clinical Excellence (NICE) (2005) Lung Cancer. *The Diagnosis and Treatment of Lung Cancer. Clinical Guideline 24*. NICE, London.

Nezu, K., Kushibe, K., Tojo, T., Takahama, M. and Kitamura, S. (1998) Recovery and limitation of exercise capacity after lung resection for lung cancer. *Chest*, **113** (6), 1511-1516.

NHS (2009) *National Lung Cancer Audit. Key Findings about the Quality of Care for People with Lung Cancer in England and Wales Incorporating Headline and Completeness from Scotland. Report for the audit period* 2007. NHS, London.

NHS Executive (1998) *Guidance on Commissioning Cancer Services: Improving Outcomes in Lung Cancer*. Department of Health, London.

Nugent, A.M., Steele, I.C. and Carragher, A.M. (1999) Effect of thoracotomy and lung resection on exercise capacity on patients with lung cancer. *Thorax*, **54**, 334-338.

O'Driscoll, M., Corner, J. and Bailey, C. (1999) The experience of breathlessness in lung cancer. *European Journal of Cancer Care*, **8**, 37-43.

Osse, B., Vernooij-Dassen, M., Schade, E. and Grol, R. (2006) Problems experienced by the informal care-givers of cancer patients and their needs for support. *Cancer Nursing*, **29** (5), 378-388.

Payne, S., Smith, P. and Dean, S. (1999) Identifying the concerns of informal carers in palliative care. *Palliative Medicine*, **13** (1), 37-45.

Plant, H.J. (2000) Living with cancer. *Understanding the Experiences of Close Relatives of People with Cancer*. Unpublished PhD thesis. University of London.

Plant, H., Sherwin, A., Moore, S., Medina, J., Ream, E. and Richardson, A. (2006) *Developing and Evaluating a Supportive Nursing Intervention for Family Members of People with Lung Cancer*. Kings College London. Available at http://www.kcl.ac.uk/teares/nmvc/external/docs/developing_evaluating.pdf. Accessed 21 October 2009.

Piper, B., Lindsay, D. and Dodd, M. (1987) Fatigue mechanisms in cancer patients: developing a nursing theory. *Oncology Nursing Forum*, **14**, 17-23.

Potter, J. and Higginson, I.J. (2004) Pain experienced by lung cancer patients: a review of prevalence, causes and pathophysiology. *Lung Cancer*, **43** (3), 247-257.

Ramalingham, S. and Balani, C. (2002) Meaningful survival in lung cancer patients *Seminars in Oncology*, **29** (1 Suppl. 4), 125-131.

Richardson, A., Halliday, D. and Wilson-Barnett, J. (2002) *Evaluating the Impact of Introducing Lung and Colorectal Nurse Specialists into the South East London Cancer Network*. King's College, University of London. Available at http://www.kcl.ac.uk/content/1/c6/02/97/19/BriefingPaperonComparativeEvaluation.pdf. Accessed 21 October 2009.

Richardson, A., Medina, J., Brown, V. and Sitzia, J. (2007a) Patients' needs assessment in cancer care: a review of assessment tools. *Supportive Care in Cancer*, **15**, 1125-1144.

Richardson, A., Plant, H., Moore, S., Medina, J., Cornwall, A. and Ream, E. (2007b) Developing supportive care for family members of people with lung cancer: a feasibility study. *Supportive Care in Cancer*, **15** (11), 1259-1269.

Rowell, N.P. and Gleeson, F.V. (2001) Steroids, radiotherapy, chemotherapy and stents for superior vena caval obstruction in carcinoma of the bronchus. *Cochrane Database of Systematic Reviews*, Issue 4, Art. No. CD001316. doi: 10.1002/14651858.CD001316.

Ryan, L. (1996) Psychosocial issues and lung cancer: a behavioural approach *Seminars in Oncology Nursing*, **12** (4), 285-294.

Sarna, L. (1998) Effectiveness of structured nursing assessment of symptom distress in advanced lung cancer. *Oncology Nursing Forum*, **25** (6), 1041-1046.

Sarna, L., Padilla, G., Holmes, C., Tashkin, D., Brecht, M.L. and Evangelista, L. (2002) Quality of life of long-term survivors of non-small-cell lung cancer. *Journal of Clinical Oncology*, **20** (13), 2920-2929.

Sarna, L., Brown, J.K., Cooley, M.E., *et al.* (2005) Quality of life and meaning of illness of women with lung cancer. *Oncology Nursing Forum*, **32** (1), E9-E19.

Schwartzstein, R.M., Lahive, K., Pope, A. and Weinberger, S.E. (1987) Cold facial stimulation reduces breathlessness induced normal subjects. *American Review of Respiratory Diseases*, **136**, 58-61.

Scottish Executive (2001) *Cancer in Scotland: Action for Change*. NHS, Scotland.

SIGN (2005) *Management of Patients with Lung Cancer. A National Clinical Guideline*. SIGN, Edinburgh.

SIGN (2008) *Control of Pain in Adults with Cancer: A National Clinical Guideline*. SIGN, Edinburgh.

Steele, R. and Fitch, M. (2008) Why patients with lung cancer do not want help with some needs. *Supportive Care in Cancer*, **16**, 251–259.

Thomas, C., Morris, S.M. and Harman, J.C. (2002) Companions through cancer: the care given by informal carers in cancer contexts. *Social Science and Medicine*, **54** (4), 529–544.

Trevatt, P. and Leary, A. (2009) A census of the advanced and specialist cancer nursing workforce in England, Northern Ireland and Wales. *European Journal of Oncology*, **14** (1), 68. doi 10.1016/j.ejon.2009.08.005.

Uchitomi, Y., Mikami, I., Nagai, K., Nishiwaki, Y., Akechi, T. and Okamura, H. (2003) Depression and psychological distress in patients during the year after curative resection of non-small-cell lung cancer. *Journal of Clinical Oncology*, **21** (1), 69–77.

White, J. (2006) Developing a nurse-led protocol for lung cancer. *Cancer Nursing Practice*, **5** (2), 31–34.

WHO (1986) *WHO's Pain Ladder*. World Health Organisation, Geneva. Available at http://www.who.int/cancer/palliative/painladder/en/. Accessed 20 October 2009.

Zabora, J., BrintzenhofeSzoc, K., Curbow, B., *et al.* (2001) The prevalence of psychological distress by cancer site. *Psycho-oncology*, **10**, 19–28.

Zieren, H.U., Muller, J.M. and Hamberger, U. (1996) Quality of life after surgical therapy of bronchogenic carcinoma. *European Journal of Cardiothoracic Surgery*, **10**, 233–237.

Chapter 7

Supportive Care in Lung Cancer

Kay Eaton

Key points

- Cancer care needs to be holistic and individualised.
- Cancer care is most effectively delivered by multidisciplinary teams.
- Good communication skills underpin all elements of care.
- Patients are central to service development.
- Cancer care is complex and negotiating care can be challenging for patients and carers - this causes suffering.

Introduction

Recent government guidance in the UK has highlighted the need for health care and social care professionals to improve the supportive care of patients with a cancer diagnosis. The provision of information and support to cancer patients is a national priority and this has been central to national policy for over 15 years, as stated in the NHS Cancer Plan (Department of Health (DH) 2000), the NICE Guidance on Improving Supportive and Palliative Care for Adults with Cancer (NICE 2004) and the Cancer Reform Strategy (DH 2007), and it is well recognised that the diagnosis and treatment of cancer can have a devastating impact on the quality of the patient's life and that of their families, friends and carers. One key aim of the NHS Cancer Plan (DH 2000) was 'to ensure that people with cancer get the right professional support and care as well as the best treatment'; other key aims were to improve the quality of life of cancer patients, to develop a patient-centred approach to care and to develop the quality of cancer services by investing in the workforce, research and development.

Lung Cancer: A Multidisciplinary Approach, First Edition. Edited by Alison Leary.
© 2012 Blackwell Publishing Ltd. Published 2012 by Blackwell Publishing Ltd.

Patients' experience of cancer care and treatment has improved over the past few years and each year more people will be alive having had a diagnosis of cancer (The National Cancer Survivorship Initiative Vision (DH 2010)). These people have very different and individual levels of need and support and there is more we can do to support and empower patients.

This chapter highlights some of the domains of supportive care for people affected by lung cancer.

Supportive care

Supportive care is an umbrella term for all services, both generalist and specialist, that may be required to support patients who are diagnosed with cancer and their carers.

Supportive care aims to provide information and emotional and practical support to enable patients and family members to adapt to and cope with the effects of the disease and any treatments given (NCHSPCS 2002; NICE 2004). Within the NHS new models of care with emphasis on partnership working between health professionals and also between health professionals and the public/patients are being designed and there is an emphasis on delivering cancer services locally as far as possible and more patients being treated in the out-patient setting. The patient's care is shared between a range of specialists and the primary care team and is based in secondary or tertiary care.

Cancer health care professionals working within the cancer networks have been developing effective coordination across care boundaries to organise and deliver cancer care based on meeting the needs and expectations of patients rather than the needs of services. It is widely acknowledged that multiprofessional teams afford the best way of providing a seamless service to cancer patients as they offer greater opportunity for coordinated care, effective communication, education, research and service development (Cole *et al.* 2000; Cheville 2001; DeLisa 2001; Santiago-Palmer and Payne 2001). Using the expertise of colleagues from other disciplines and specialities can facilitate optimal patient outcomes across organisational boundaries in the care pathway.

Putting the individual patient's needs higher on the agenda is important and this is implicit in the Cancer Reform Strategy (DH 2007) and the National Cancer Survivorship Initiative Vision (DH 2010) and in endeavouring to provide a supportive care culture. Whatever the health care setting, patients and their carers should have the central role in each step along the care pathway. In essence, we have a great deal of evidence telling us what patients would like and need, and with the skills, knowledge, expertise, communication and willing collaboration of health care professionals, we have the potential to greatly improve the quality of patient care and the well-being of people affected by cancer.

Communicating the 'diagnosis'

Today many more people are surviving cancer and living longer with a diagnosis of cancer. This is a result of earlier diagnosis and improvement in treatment of the disease, but unfortunately there are still delays in patient presentation that can result in more advanced disease at diagnosis and consequently poorer patient outcomes (case for change). Lung cancer remains the most common cause of cancer death in men and women in the United Kingdom. Lung cancer therefore has a serious impact not only on the health of patients and on their family and friends but on the nation as well. It was estimated for the year 2008 that there were 63522 patients living in the United Kingdom with a lung cancer diagnosis (Maddams et al. 2009).

It is not surprising that the diagnosis and treatment of cancer are known to be associated with high levels of psychological distress (Derogatis et al. 1983; Folkman and Greer 2000) and especially around the time of diagnosis. The literature has shown that the way in which the diagnosis of cancer is communicated to the patient and family is crucial. If it is done badly it can have a long-lasting effect on the patient, it is not likely to be forgotten, and it can set the tone for the ongoing relationship of the patient with the doctor and the multiprofessional team.

Good communication skills of the health professional are essential; however, there is evidence to show that the breaking of bad news may not be done very well. Evidence has shown that the communication skills of health care professionals can be improved by training, and those who have undergone advanced communications skills training that included 'breaking bad news' have been shown to have better outcomes in terms of patient satisfaction and in terms of the anxiety and depression that patients experience in the long term.

There is no evidence that honest communication causes detrimental effects to the patient (Dein 2006, p. 59). Fallowfield (1997) found that health care professionals often censor their information-giving in an attempt to protect patients from potentially hurtful or sad news; Fallowfield states that this shielding can cause difficulties to the patient. Attitudes towards informing patients of a cancer diagnosis or that they have a terminal illness have changed since the 1970s. In the USA and Europe it is presumed generally that patients should be informed of their diagnosis. However, in some other countries, it is still common for the diagnosis of cancer to be concealed from the patient, especially a terminal illness. There is therefore a need for health care professionals to have knowledge of the different cultural patterns of communication among the populations in which they work. Patients need information given in a clear and sensitive way and in language they understand.

There is evidence to support the view that the majority of patients want honest communication to allow them to make informed decisions about treatment options and other important issues that may radically affect or alter their future lives.

For many patients with a diagnosis of lung cancer, being given the information that their future care will have a palliative focus rather than one that strives for a cure can be devastating and can rob the patient of 'hope' for their future. It can mean their personal view of their future has been taken away and altered forever. It is important that in such circumstances, although a guarantee of a cure cannot be given, the health care professional should make it clear that they will try to make sure that everything possible will be done for the patient's well-being and their individual needs and concerns will be addressed.

Recognising the emotional impact of cancer, it is essential that people affected by cancer at the time of diagnosis have individualised information, advice and specialist support to help them to cope with cancer from the time cancer is suspected through the subsequent stages of the disease. Patients vary in the extent to which they wish to be involved in the information and decision-making process. It is for the clinician caring for the patient to elicit the wishes of the patient.

As a result of medical advancement we are now seeing increased use of treatment regimens that combine radiotherapy and chemotherapy. It is predicted that this will be associated with improved rates of survival but it can result in increased side effects associated with treatment. Patients with cancer are now being actively treated later in the disease trajectory and patients and families should be offered opportunities to be fully informed of the implications of both the disease and the treatment. The time required for this will vary from patient to patient. All health care interventions should have the long-term interests of patients as the focal point whether they are undergoing active treatment or supportive and palliative care. Whatever the situation, the principles of care remain the same and are centred on the importance of good and meaningful communication with patient and family, providing appropriate care, care that is focused on improving the patients' well-being and responding to the ongoing and changing needs of patients, both physical and psychological.

Attitudes towards cancer

Despite recent advances in the treatment of cancer, generally cancer is the disease most people fear most. Cultural factors influence the understanding of attitudes towards cancer. Social attitudes with regard to cancer are highly variable across different cultural groups. An individual's attitudes can be shaped from personal life experiences of friends and family, previous illness, hospital experiences, cancer stories in the media and hearsay. Attitudes of fear related to cancer are widespread and cancer is a subject about which few people can think without emotion and concern. People generally tend to have a pessimistic outlook toward cancer when a diagnosis of cancer is made. Patients can be fearful about the loss of an expected future and not being able to plan their life far ahead. Today we live in a future-orientated society, which does not help matters.

Cassells (2004) says that it is not the cancer but all the multiple meanings placed into the future associated with a diagnosis of cancer that people find so difficult, and this is described in the literature as a threat/loss situation. Suffering varies from person to person and people can be devoid of physical pain or symptoms but suffer from what they feel they have lost, which is connected to part of the person's cultural belief, values and life experiences.

Some of the patient's fears may be about:

- Loss of body parts
- Mutilation
- Loss of self-worth
- Fear of treatment
- Loss of control
- Fear of pain
- Fear of death/painful death

Recognising the losses is important and a listening presence to the individual's suffering is often welcomed.

Uncertainty

Uncertainty is also a main concern of patients diagnosed with cancer. Difficulties and delays in reaching a diagnosis are not uncommon and this can be a very concerning time for patients and families which should not be underestimated. There can be uncertainty of the diagnosis initially, with the waiting for results of diagnostic investigation. Following on from the diagnostic phase, there is the uncertainty of treatment modality and the side effects of treatment. In the longer term there is the uncertainty whether the cancer treatment will be successful and cure or control the cancer, and what the prognosis will be after treatment has been completed. It appears from the literature that the uncertainty does not disappear, and many disease-free cancer survivors experience anxiety over the possibility of a cancer recurrence (Lee-Jones and Humphries 1997). Cancer can be summarised as a complex disease that does not follow a straightforward course and many patients find this difficult to adjust to. Some patients will need help to cope with feelings of vulnerability and the uncertainty of life.

Cassells (2004) states that 'to be successful in treating the sickness and alleviating suffering, doctors must know more about the sick person and the illness than just the name of the disease and the science that explains it'. Cassells is stating the importance of assessment and in communicating effectively with our patients. This means understanding how the illness affects the patient individually, how it affects their lives and how it is continuing to affect them. Knowing the subjective dimension of illness is essential and being a supportive presence and using active listening is as important as talking. Eliciting from the patient what they are feeling and what their concerns and needs are at regular intervals – as their needs can and will change over time – is a major part of cancer care.

Psychological distress

Patients diagnosed with cancer will suffer some degree of stress and anxiety. This is true no matter what the diagnosis or prognosis, but the prevalence of psychological distress among cancer patients is difficult to estimate and reports vary depending on the diagnostic tools and criteria used in the studies. Patients diagnosed and treated for cancer have an increased risk of developing anxiety and depression (Derogatis *et al*. 1983; Folkman and Greer 2000; Nicholson-Perry and Burgess 2002). In a large study of patients with different cancer types, the prevalence of psychological distress and variations in distress showed that lung cancer patients had higher levels of distress (43.4% compared with around 30% in the general cancer population). Fallowfield (2001) found in a large study in the UK that 36% of patient with various cancers were suffering from clinically significant distress. Research studies claim that the poor prognosis and self-attribution associated with smoking may be a contributing factor in the increased level of distress in persons with lung cancer (Zabora *et al*. 2001; Walker *et al*. 2006).

Patients with cancer tend to have a high frequency of depressive symptoms, varying from 4.5% to over 50% in different settings and for different cancers. Key points of psychological and emotional vulnerability include the time of a cancer diagnosis, the treatment end points and episodes of disease recurrence. The incidence of depression increases with advanced disease, physical debilitation, pain and other symptoms experienced by the patient.

Patients most at risk of developing psychological problems in response to cancer include those with a previous history of psychological disturbance, those with little or no social support, those who experience stressful life events of a severe kind in addition to having cancer, and those with certain coping styles such as:

- Anxious preoccupation
- Helplessness/hopelessness
- A stoic acceptance of their fate

(Greer *et al*. 1979).

The recognition of depression and other psychological and psychiatric disorders in patients with cancer is generally poor and clinically significant distress often goes unnoticed by cancer professionals (Sollner *et al*. 2001).

Inadequate diagnosis of depression in cancer patients can cause reduction in their quality of life. It could also interfere with their ability to make important treatment decisions, and to persevere with a prescribed course of cancer treatment.

Good psychological support services should be available to support patients from the point of diagnosis onwards. There is fairly good evidence that psychosocial interventions are effective in reducing distress and promoting adjustment of patients with cancer. In some cases psychosocial intervention may also reduce the severity of physical symptoms experienced by the patient.

There are many factors influencing the social relationships of the person with a cancer diagnosis. In the society we live in today, with high levels of divorce and single-person families, the 'extended family' is rarely present, and therefore social support for the patient may be limited. Patients can feel isolated because of the cancer diagnosis and can feel that cancer can be regarded as a 'taboo' subject, unlike other illnesses, because of cultural norms or as a consequence of public misconception of cancer being contagious. The association of cancer with death can bring fear, anxiety and stigma and can alter family dynamics or social networks. A diagnosis of cancer can bring significant challenges to patients in their daily activities, work and social relationships.

People can be prone to make moral judgements on lung cancer sufferers, appear to lack the capacity for empathy and blame smokers for getting lung cancer (i.e. 'they brought it on themselves'). It is apparent from social support research that emotional support from relationships reduces the impact of life stressors such as illness (Wills 1992). The number and significance of stressors both directly and indirectly related to cancer in a patient's life are important factors in determining the degree of adjustment. These will vary according to stage and treatment of a person's cancer. Patients' uncertainties and fears increase their need for support and the fear and stigma associated with disease can create isolation and communication problems that can lead to a decrease in their access to social support.

In the literature, hope appears to be crucial to a person's physical, psychosocial and spiritual well-being. Having hope is important to the patient and the family and perhaps no-one is more aware of the need for hope than the person with a diagnosis of cancer. Generally the patient hopes the treatment will be successful, hopes for recovery, and hopes for survival. Without hope, patients can have feelings of helplessness and depression, which can lead to social isolation, feelings of abandonment and uncertainties regarding often long-held spiritual or religious beliefs.

Weisman and Worden (1976) have identified the hundred days after diagnosis as a time when patients become concerned with the meaning of life, death and illness. This is a time when the patient can be vulnerable and struggling to cope with the diagnosis. Patients can feel a need to employ spiritual coping strategies and a search for meaning in their lives.

So how does one help to promote hope? This can be difficult as any information given, regarding prognosis for example, needs to be grounded in a realistic context. Actively listening, eliciting and hearing concerns can help, together with offering information when appropriate. Patients may be reluctant to share their concerns, anxieties or worries about the future with their families/friends in order to avoid presenting themselves as a burden to others but will often open up to a health care professional.

Fincham *et al.* (2005) found in their study that an important issue for cancer patients was the opportunity to develop a relationship with a key health care professional during their illness. A familiar key contact person was preferred rather than seeing different members of staff at each hospital visit, and this is especially important when patients have little social or psychological support of their own.

It may be appropriate for the patient to be offered referral to a cancer counsellor or clinical psychologist to help them cope with the impact of their disease on their lives.

A family-centred approach to care

A family-centred approach to care is important as lung cancer is a disease that is generally characterised by rapid physical deterioration and an earlier than expected death. There will be complexity of patient needs, physical and psychosocial, and an ongoing comprehensive assessment will need to be made by the health care professionals involved to elicit individual patient concerns, to provide optimal symptom management and referral to appropriate health and social care.

Family members/caregivers are often an important communication link between the patient and health care professionals and especially when the patient becomes unwell or when communication barriers exist. It is important also to consider the needs and concerns of family members as they are central to the care of the patient and need to be considered as a whole.

There is much in the literature regarding the impact of a cancer diagnosis in the family, but in practice it appears that the impact of cancer on a family can be underestimated and a neglected area. We know that family members of patients with cancer can often feel unsupported by health services (Plant *et al.* 2000; Krishnasamy and Wilkie 2001).

A diagnosis of cancer can be very difficult for relatives to accept and cope with. In some relationships, the development of cancer in one of the partners can strengthen the relationship, while in others it can have a negative effect. As previously mentioned, a cancer diagnosis for a family member can disrupt family life and their expectations and plans for the future and they can move from feeling secure and stable into instability (Plant 1995). This will have an effect on the entire family. Primarily, family members or carers have to manage the patient's response to the illness and also their own psychological reactions, which they may be reluctant to voice. The carers' concerns can often take second place and be neglected. Health care providers tend to focus on the patient, but caring can be emotionally and physically tiring. It is important to see therefore that their concerns should also be of concern to the health care professional, especially if they have little social or psychological support of their own. Nurses should try to elicit the concerns of the carer from an emotional and practical point of view and offer them information on where they can find support. Patients and carers should be given support and information including, if required, access to welfare rights and benefits advice and information regarding self-help and patient/carer support groups. Practical support may be required such as domestic help, transport, child care and advocacy and befriending schemes.

Health care professionals can sometimes offer an alternative perspective to a problem or concern and can offer advice on such matters as lifestyle modification and stress management and help the patient to mobilise their own coping strategies.

Family members and caregivers may have inadequate knowledge, skills or preparation for the assessment and care of often very complex symptoms that the patient may be suffering from, particularly in advanced malignant disease. Krishnasamy (1996) described family members needing and wanting information and advice primarily in the following areas:

- Personal care, comfort and support needs of the patient
- Communication issues
- Nutritional advice and how to get patients to eat
- Coping with decreased energy
- Worries about how to deal with an emergency situation
- Symptom relief/management (Kristjanson et al. 1998).

Often when patients are undergoing chemotherapy and/or radiotherapy for their cancer treatment they can struggle physically and emotionally. The symptoms of both the disease and its treatment are often managed by family caregivers at home. Support, information and educational intervention for acquiring the necessary knowledge and skills should be provided for family caregivers to help them to feel more confident within the home situation. They need to be aware of the significance associated with symptoms and the often simple interventions and care that can be used to provide relief and comfort in the home environment.

Improving the patient experience: care across the pathway

Care and treatment of the patient with cancer invariably involves multiple providers of health care in many care settings and often requires the patient to travel from one cancer treatment centre or unit to another. Some patients will previously have had minimal contact with the health care system and its complexities and they can find it confusing.

There is a strong relationship between socioeconomic deprivation and incidence of lung cancer. However, Bennett et al. (2008) show in their study that a diagnosis of adenocarcinoma is less strongly related to deprivation than lung cancer of other histological types. London and other major cities are recognised as having a significant number of deprived communities and research has identified a link between deprivation and poorer outcomes from treatment and lowered life expectancy and, for the majority of cancers, patients from the most deprived areas have worse survival rates. The cultural diversity of inner cities requires services to be delivered in a culturally appropriate and sensitive manner, with particular attention paid to the needs of black and ethnic minority groups and those vulnerable through mental health problems, learning disabilities, deprivation and sexual orientation (Action for London Working Group 2007). It is a challenge, and cancer services require the flexibility to identify, acknowledge and support a particularly wide range of needs of patients.

Patients with lung cancer often live with advanced cancer that is incurable and many undergo multiple cancer treatments with palliative intent with the aim of trying to contain the disease progression. Patients can experience several concurrent symptoms associated with the disease and treatment, and the type and number of symptoms may vary and change as the patient moves through the phases of the illness. Thorough and accurate symptom assessment of the patient provides an effective way of identifying and monitoring specific patient problems and a way of evaluating treatment and intervention. We know that people with lung cancer suffer from concurrent severe symptoms such as fatigue, pain, anorexia, coughing and insomnia that have an adverse impact on quality of life (Cooley *et al.* 2003; Chen and Tseng 2006; Hoffman *et al.* 2007). The three most common and severe symptoms reported as affecting patients with a lung cancer diagnosis are pain, fatigue and insomnia.

In a large study, Jiong and Girgis (2006) looked at the unmet needs of lung cancer patients compared with groups of patients with breast cancer and prostate cancer. The mean number of needs of patients with lung cancer were significantly higher than in other cancer patients: 53.4% had concerns about their family members or those close to them; 52% had fears about the cancer spreading; 49% had fears about physical disability; 53.3% were afraid of not being able to do things they used to do; 48% experienced lack of energy and tiredness; and 38.8% experienced pain.

Cooley (2000) found that, compared with other major cancers, lung cancer has more symptomatology and increased levels of anorexia and pain. Pain, dyspnoea and anorexia were found to be the most common and intense symptoms in advanced lung cancer. There is evidence of successful non-pharmacological intervention for managing the debilitating and distressing symptoms such as breathlessness, weight loss, anorexia, cachexia, depression, cough and difficulty swallowing. For some patients with advanced disease, palliative care intervention and referral to a specialist palliative care service may be appropriate. The End of Life Care Strategy centres on improving care and addressing the needs of this group of patients (DH 2008a).

There is a high prevalence of malnutrition in patients with malignant disease, thought to affect up to 80% of patients (Capra *et al.* 2001). Nutritional issues can arise from the tumour itself, treatment effects, and the patient's reaction to illness and stress. This is important as malnutrition contributes to reduced immunity, increased length of hospital stay, higher patient complication rates and treatment requirements and increased morbidity and mortality (Whitiman 1999; Finley 2000; Capra *et al.* 2001; Milne *et al.* 2003).

Cancer cachexia is characterised by prolonged and significant anorexia and body wasting and can affect approximately 50% of cancer patients (Finley 2000; Milne *et al.* 2003). Unintentional, significant weight loss is detrimental to all cancer patients including the overweight and obese (Whitiman 1999). Early and regular nutritional screening is vital to identify and manage a cancer patient's nutritional risk. Timely referral to a qualified dietician and dietetic intervention are important in the prevention and management of weight loss and have been shown to improve patient outcomes (Capra *et al.* 2001; Milne *et al.* 2003).

We know from the literature that patients with lung cancer can suffer from a high frequency of symptoms. It should be remembered that patients do not always independently report their symptoms and there may be several reasons for this. Therefore, the primary responsibility for undertaking a holistic needs assessment including assessment of symptoms must rest with the health care professional. The Clinical Nurse Specialist has an important role in recognising and addressing unmet needs in his or her patients and acting as advocate for patients and families, and can offer support or referrals to relevant health care professionals to help address these needs. For example, in the case of dyspnoea, it is not uncommon for there to be contributing factors such as anaemia and cachexia, which can be treated accordingly if recognised.

As mentioned earlier, family caregivers are an important communication link between health care professionals and the patient. This can be especially important when patients are too unwell or weak to convey their feelings, or have difficulty in recalling their symptoms accurately.

It is important to highlight the supportive and therapeutic role of the Lung Cancer Clinical Nurse Specialist (CNS). It is recognised that the CNS has a valuable role and the supportive and coordinating function of the Clinical Nurse Specialist is important throughout the entire care pathway, and especially so at the diagnostic stage and in the follow-up phase after treatment has been completed. At present there is limited evidence available on the needs of cancer patients who have finished treatment but there is some literature that does indicate that this is a very stressful period for patients and that developing a post-treatment plan of care can be helpful as patient care does not end when treatment ends. It is clear that suffering is common across all phases of the cancer pathway and is individualised and personal. Often patients are feeling worse, for example, at the end of a course of treatment when side effects of treatment can be at their maximum. Nicholson and Wells (2003) state that patients at this stage are in no-man's land, 'not actually sick, nor are they well, neither healthy nor cured and they may be suffering from side effects of treatment'. When treatment is finished or stopped it is a difficult time; patients can experience feelings of abandonment and can be left wondering whether treatment has been successful or whether there will be a recurrence of the disease. C.S. Lewis in *A Grief Observed* comments that 'life and also grief can be considered akin to a type of waiting … hanging about waiting for something to happen. It gives life a permanently provisional feeling. It doesn't seem worth doing anything'.

Some patients will want to know their prognosis, but prognostic prediction is difficult. There is evidence that health care professionals are generally poor at predicting prognosis in the last year of the patient's life – with errors 30% of the time, and two-thirds of these being over-optimistic (Glare *et al.* 2003).

Not all patients want to discuss issues regarding prognosis or planning ahead for end-of-life care, but they should have the opportunity to do so, as the lack of opportunity can have implications that affect quality of life for the patient and also for the family.

Summary

The effects of cancer and its treatment can have a devastating effect on the patient's daily life and quality of life for them and their family, and no two patients have the same needs or concerns. It is important for all health care professionals to hear the individual patient's personal experiences. Full holistic assessment of an individual patient's needs at key stages in the care pathway is essential so that the issues and challenges associated with the disease and its treatment, the physical, psychological, social and spiritual needs of patient care can be identified and addressed. This will allow professionals, patients, family and carers to work together in a coordinated approach with the aim of providing appropriate supportive care, easing suffering and improving the quality of life for the patient.

References

Action for London Working Group (2007) *Action for London: A Vision for Cancer Care in the Capital 2007–2010*. Network Nurse Directors Group & Macmillan Cancer Support London.

Bennett, V.A., Davies, E.A., Jack, R.H., Mak, V. and Moller, H. (2008) Histological subtype of lung cancer in relation to socio-economic deprivation in South East England. *BMC Cancer*, **8**, 139.

Capra, S., Ferguson, M. and Reid, K. (2001) Cancer: impact of nutrition intervention outcome – nutrition issues for patients. *Nutrition*, **17**, 769–772.

Cassells, E.J. (2004) *The Nature of Suffering and the Goals of Medicine*, 2nd edn. Oxford University Press, Oxford.

Chen, M.L. and Tseng, H.C. (2006) Symptom clusters in cancer patients. *Supportive Care in Cancer*, **14**, 825–830.

Cheville, A. (2001) Rehabilitation of patients with advanced cancer. *Cancer Supplement*, **92** (4), 1039–1048.

Cole, R.P., Scialla, S.J. and Lucien, B. (2000) Functional recovery in cancer rehabilitations. *Archives of Physical Medicine and Rehabilitation*, **81**, 623–627.

Cooley, M.E. (2000) Symptoms in adults with lung cancer: a systematic research review. *Journal of Pain and Symptom Management*, **19**, 137–153.

Cooley, M.E., Short, T.H., Moriarty, H.J., *et al.* (2003) Symptom prevalence, distress and change over time in adults receiving treatment for lung cancer. *Psycho-oncology*, **12** (7), 694–708.

Dein, S. (2006) *Culture and Cancer Care. Anthropological Insights in Oncology*. Open University Press, Buckingham.

DeLisa, J.A. (2001) A history of cancer rehabilitation. *Cancer*, **92**, 975-979.

DH (2000) *The NHS Cancer Plan. A Plan for Investment. A Plan for Reform*. HMSO, London.

DH (2007) *Cancer Reform Strategy*. HMSO, London.

DH (2008a) *End of Life Care Strategy*. HMSO, London.

DH (2008) *NHS Next Stage Review Final Report - High Quality Care for All*. HMSO, London.

DH (2010) *National Cancer Survivorship Initiative Vision*. HMSO, London.

Derogatis, L.R., Morrow, G.R., Fetting, J., *et al*. (1983) The prevalence of psychiatric disorders among cancer patients. *Journal of the American Medical Association*, **249**, 751-757.

Fallowfield, L. (1997) Truth sometimes hurts but deceit hurts more. *Annals of the New York Academy of Sciences*, **809**, 525-536.

Fallowfield, L., Ratcliffe, D., Jenkins, V. and Saul, J. (2001) Psychiatric morbidity and its recognition by doctors in patients with cancer. *British Journal of Cancer*, **84** (8), 1011-1015.

Finley, J.P. (2000) Management of cancer cachexia. *Advanced Practice in Acute Critical Care Clinical* **11** (4), 590-603.

Fincham, L., Copp, G., Caldwell, K., Jones, L. and Tookman, A. (2005) Supportive care: experience of cancer patients. *European Journal of Oncology Nursing*, **9** (3), 258-268.

Folkman, S. and Greer, S. (2000) Promoting psychological wellbeing in the face of serious illness: when theory, research and practice inform each other. *Psycho-oncology*, **9**, 11-19.

Glare, P., Kiran, V., Jones, M., *et al*. (2003) A systematic review of physicians' survival predictions in terminally ill cancer patients. *British Medical Journal*, **327**, 195.

Greer, S., Morris, T. and Pettingale, K.W. (1979) Psychological response to breast cancer: effect on outcome. *Lancet*, **2** (8146), 785-787.

Hoffman, A.J., Given, B.A., Von Eye, A., *et al*. (2007) Relationships among pain, fatigue, insomnia and gender with persons with lung cancer. *Oncology Nursing Forum*, **34** (4), 785-792.

Jiong, L.I. and Girgis, A.F. (2006) Supportive care needs: are patients with lung cancer a neglected population? *Psycho-oncology*, **15**, 509-516.

Krishnasamy, M. (1996) Social support and the patient: a consideration of the literature. *Journal of Advanced Nursing*, **23** (4), 757-762.

Krishnasamy, M., Wilkie, E., *et al*. (2001) Lung cancer healthcare needs assessment: patients' and informal carers' responses to a national mail questionnaire survey. *Palliative Medicine*, **15** (3), 213-227.

Kristjanson, L.L., Nikoletti, S., Porock, D., Smith, M., Lobchuk, M. and Pedler, P. (1998) Congruence between patients' and family caregivers' perceptions of symptom distress in patients with terminal cancer. *Journal of Palliative Care*, **14**, 24-32.

Lee-Jones, C., Humphris, G., Dixon, R. and Hatcher, M.B. (1997) Fear of cancer recurrence, a literature review and proposed cognitive formulation to explain exacerbation of recurrence fears. *Psycho-oncology*, **6** (2), 95-105.

Lewis, C.S. (1961) *A Grief Observed*. Faber, London.

Maddams, J., Brewster, A., Gavin, A., *et al*. (2009) Cancer prevalence in the United Kingdom: estimates for 2008. *British Journal of Cancer*, **101**, 541-547.

Milne, A.C., Potter, J. and Avenell, A. (2003) *Protein and Energy Supplementation in Elderly People at Risk from Malnutrition*. (Cochrane Review). Cochrane Library, Issue 3. Oxford: Update Software.

NCHSPCS (2002) *Definitions of Supportive and Palliative Care: a Consultation Paper*. National Council for Hospice and Specialist Palliative Care Services, London.

NICE (2004). *Improving Supportive and Palliative Care for Adults with Cancer*. National Institute for Clinical Excellence, London.

Nicholson, C. and Wells, M. (2003) After treatment is over. In: *Supportive Care in Radiotherapy* (eds S. Faithfull and M. Wells). Churchill Livingstone, Edinburgh.

Nicholson Perry, K. and Burgess, M. (2002) *Communication in Cancer Care*. Blackwell, Oxford.

Plant, H. (1995) The expenses of families of newly diagnosed cancer patients – selected findings. In: *Nursing Research in Cancer Care* (eds A. Richardson and J. Wilson-Barnett). Scutari Press, London.

Plant, H., Bredin, M., Krishnasamy, M. and Corner, J. (2000) Working with resistance, tension and objectivity: conducting a randomised trial of a nursing intervention for breathlessness. *NT Research*, **5** (6), 426–433.

Santiago-Palmer, J. and Payne, R. (2001) Palliative care and rehabilitation. *Cancer* **92** (4), 1049–1052.

Sollner, W., De Vries, A. and Steixner, E., *et al.* (2001) How successful are oncologists in identifying patient distress, perceived social support, and need for psychosocial counselling? *British Journal of Cancer*, **84** (2), 197–185.

Walker, M.S., Zona, D.M. and Fisher, E.B. (2006) Depressive symptoms after lung cancer surgery: their relation to coping style and social support. *Psycho-oncology*, **15**, 684–693.

Weisman, A.D. and Worden J.W. (1976) *Coping and Vulnerability in Cancer Patients. Final Report*. National Cancer Institute, Bethesda, MD.

Whitiman, M.M. (1999) The starving patient: supportive care for people with cancer. *Clinical Journal of Oncology Nursing*, **4** (3), 121–125.

Wills, T.A. (1992) The helping process in the context of personal relationships. In: *Helping and Being Helped – Naturistic Studies*. SAGE Publications, London.

Zabora, J., Brintzenhofeszoe, K., Curbow, B., *et al.* (2001) The prevalence of psychological distress by cancer site. *Psycho-oncology*, **10**, 19–28.

Chapter 8
End of Life Care

Michael Coughlan

Key points

- Palliative care is an approach that improves the quality of life of patients and their families facing the problems associated with life-threatening illness.
- Lung cancer patients are likely to present with advanced disease.
- Many health care professionals still see dying as a failure of health care rather than part of a natural process.
- Good symptom control is vital in end of life care.

Introduction

While some patients with lung cancer will benefit from active treatment (Souhami and Tobias 2005), the majority of patients present with relatively advanced disease (NHS Executive 1998), and in England the disease has one of the lowest survival outcomes of any cancer, with only 6.5% of men and 7.6% of women surviving 5 years in the period 1999–2003 (National Statistics 2007). It is estimated that lung cancer accounts for over 35 000 deaths each year in the UK (Cancer Research UK 2011), a statistic that challenges health care professionals to meet the demand for good end of life care.

Palliative and end of life care

Modern end of life care has its roots in the hospice movement, and Dame Cicely Saunders, who trained first as a nurse then as a doctor, is credited with being the founder of the modern hospice movement. She developed the principles of modern palliative care, characterised by a systematic approach to symptom

Lung Cancer: A Multidisciplinary Approach, First Edition. Edited by Alison Leary.
© 2012 Blackwell Publishing Ltd. Published 2012 by Blackwell Publishing Ltd.

management, through research conducted at St Joseph's Hospice in East London in the late 1950s (Pennell and Corner 2001; Winslow and Clark 2005).

The National Council for Palliative Care (2006a) emphasises the importance of being clear about what is meant by the term 'end of life care' and proposes the following definition: 'the provision of supportive and palliative care in response to the assessed needs of patient and family during the last phase of life' (p. 3). Thus it is a clearly defined stage of the palliative care continuum, which in previous decades might have been referred to less sensitively as the 'terminal phase'.

The World Health Organization (WHO 2002) offers a comprehensive definition of palliative care that identifies several important issues that will be elaborated upon in this chapter. *Palliative care* in terms of this definition is

> an approach that improves the quality of life of patients and their families facing the problems associated with life-threatening illness, through the prevention and relief of suffering by means of early identification and impeccable assessment and treatment of pain and other problems, physical, psychosocial and spiritual.

According to the World Health Organization, *palliative care*:

- Provides relief from pain and other distressing symptoms
- Affirms life and regards dying as a normal process
- Intends neither to hasten or postpone death
- Integrates the psychological and spiritual aspects of patient care
- Offers a support system to help patients live as actively as possible until death
- Offers a support system to help the family cope during the patient's illness and in their own bereavement
- Uses a team approach to address the needs of patients and their families, including bereavement counselling, if indicated
- Will enhance quality of life, and may also positively influence the course of illness
- Is applicable early in the course of illness, in conjunction with other therapies that are intended to prolong life, such as chemotherapy or radiation therapy, and includes those investigations needed to better understand and manage distressing clinical complications.

(WHO 2002)

Dying in the twenty-first century

Despite the fact that the British Isles are the birthplace of the hospice movement, the research into symptom management conducted by Cicely Saunders and others over the last 50 years, and the fact that NICE (2004) has identified end of life care as being a 'core aspect' of care, many people still do not receive optimum care and suffer an undignified death with uncontrolled symptoms (Ellershaw 2003; Griffin *et al.* 2007). The NHS Cancer Plan (Department of Health (DH) 2000) recognised that 'too many patients still experience distressing symptoms, poor nursing care, poor psychological and social support, and inadequate communication' with professionals (p. 7).

The Healthcare Commission's report on 16 000 complaints reviewed between 2004 and 2006 found that many were concerned with the care provided to dying patients and the relationships between healthcare staff and family members following a patient's death (Healthcare Commission 2007). Furthermore, inadequate care at the end of life has significant consequences for the bereaved (DH 2000, 2008; National Council for Palliative Care 2006b).

Seymour and Ingleton (2004) identify some factors that can make caring for people at the end of life difficult in the modern age:

- Health professionals having come to regard death as a failure
- Problems diagnosing the process of dying
- Managing complex ethical dilemmas

These features, explored below, affect the clarity of our decision making and our ability to care for those approaching the end of their lives. As a result we are failing in our duty as professionals by denying patients and their partners their right to effective supportive care (Regnard and Hockley 2004).

Health professionals' attitudes to the dying

Rather than regarding dying as a normal process, many health professionals have come to regard death as a failure, a view that has serious implications for patient care (Seymour and Ingleton 2004; DH 2008).

There is a great deal of research evidence that demonstrates that professionals find caring for people with cancer – and particularly those with advanced disease – very stressful (Corner 1993; Irvine 1993; McCaughan and Parahoo 2000; Lanceley 2008) and that nurses use avoidance behaviours when caring for dying patients (Brent *et al.* 1991; Frommelt 1991; Wilkinson 1997). This situation is possibly a result of the fact that during the twentieth century dying was 'professionalized' and removed from people's everyday experience, with the majority of people now dying in institutional care settings (Clark 1993; DH 2008). At the opening of the twentieth century, around 85% of people died in their own homes, a figure that dropped to 50% by the middle of the century, and to only 18% by the early twenty-first century (DH 2008). Whereas previously people had died at home surrounded by their families and friends who knew how to relate to the dying person and manage death (Seymour and Ingleton 2004), modern society as a whole now lacks any familiarity with death (DH 2008). As a result, a 'death denying' attitude has developed within many Western societies, which has resulted in even the discussion of death being regarded as taboo (Kubler-Ross 1970; Ariès 1993; Pennell and Corner 2001; DH 2008).

It is 40 years since Kubler-Ross (1970) argued that our fear of death appeared to increase as medical science advanced, and Seymour and Ingleton (2004) suggest that our negative attitude to death has contributed to us focusing on care of the physical body to the detriment of spiritual and psycho-social dimensions of care. Indeed, the Department of Health (DH 2008) identifies society's attitude to death as a significant issue in service delivery and associates it with an inability of many health and social care professionals to discuss death and the process of dying with clients. Kubler-Ross (1970) maintains that we can effectively care for dying patients only when we overcome our fear and come to terms with our own mortality. Ellershaw and Murphy (2011) conclude that 'a major cultural shift' is needed if the needs of dying patients are to be met by professionals.

Diagnosing dying

Seymour and Ingleton (2004) explain that medical technology and new treatments not only prolong life but also make the process of dying much longer than previously. These advances also make diagnosing dying more difficult, particularly when the prevailing culture is focused on cure (Ellershaw and Murphy 2011). Failure to identify the fact that the patient is dying means that the goals of management are not reviewed, leading to inappropriate investigations and treatments being continued. Faull and Nyatanga (2005) identify the failure to review the plan of care as being probably the most important factor in not achieving a 'good death', as referrals to palliative care and other supportive services may not be made and optimum symptom control not achieved. In addition, those close to the patient are denied the opportunity to prepare, as best they can, for their inevitable loss (Hanson 2004), and instead hold onto unrealistic hopes of recovery.

While some patients deteriorate and die suddenly and unexpectedly, the National Council for Palliative Care (2006b) points out that the last days of life usually have recognisable features such as those outlined in Table 8.1 that might suggest that a patient is dying. When interpreting the significance of symptoms it is important to examine them in context, consider the overall clinical picture and identify and treat potentially reversible symptoms where possible (Regnard and Hockley 2004; Ellershaw and Murphy 2011). It is also important to remember that the process is often gradual but progressive (Faull and Nyatanga 2005).

The complexity of diagnosing dying is recognised in the most recent version of the *Liverpool Care Pathway for the Dying Patient* (Marie Curie Palliative Care Institute Liverpool 2009) – an integrated care pathway developed to improve end of life care (Ellershaw 2011). The new version has moved away from using a list of possible indicators that might be suggestive of impending death (such as those in Table 8.1), and has adopted a less prescriptive algorithm to aid decision making (Ellershaw and Murphy 2011). It is stressed that the decision that a patient might be entering the last days or hours of life

Table 8.1 Possible indicators of irreversible decline.

- Gaunt appearance
- Profound weakness
- Drowsiness
- Disorientation
- Bedbound state
- Diminished oral intake
- Unable to take tablets
- Poor concentration
- Semi-comatose state
- Skin colour changes
- Temperature change at extremities

Kinder and Ellershaw (2003); Faull and Nyatanga (2005); National Council for Palliative Care (2006b).

should be made by the multidisciplinary team (consisting of at least a doctor and nurse). The decision should be reviewed every 3 days, or if the patient's level of consciousness or functional status improve, or if anyone has expressed concern about the management plan. Any potentially reversible causes of the deterioration should be excluded and the advice of the specialist palliative care team or another second opinion sought (Marie Curie Palliative Care Institute Liverpool 2009).

Managing complex ethical dilemmas

The potential offered by recent advances in medical technology, together with our difficulties in diagnosing the process of dying, and our view that the death of our patients is a failure (DH 2008), affects the clarity of our decision making and means that we are ill-prepared to deal with the ethical dilemmas that end of life care presents. Unfortunately, decisions about the management and care of dying people are often intrinsically ethical in nature because they involve beliefs about how people should live and die (Regnard and Hockley 2004; Roy 2004).

Decisions about symptom management (particularly the use of opioids) and about stopping inappropriate or futile treatments can be particularly difficult, and are sometimes confused with euthanasia, which is the *intentional* bringing about of the death of another person, for the benefit of that person (Singleton and McLaren 1995). In euthanasia, death may be brought about either actively by administering a drug or treatment with the *intention* of hastening death, or passively by withholding or discontinuing treatments, again with the *intention* of hastening death (Thompson *et al*. 2006). This, according to many authors is quite different from allowing a *dying* person to die by discontinuing life-prolonging treatments (Roy 2004). Indeed, the World Health Organization (WHO 2002) explicitly takes a pro-life stance by stating that palliative care 'intends neither to hasten [n]or postpone death'.

Table 8.2 Suggested benefits of dehydration at the end of life.

- Reduced urine output – reduced problems with micturition/incontinence
- Decreased gastrointestinal fluid – reduced nausea and vomiting
- Reduced pulmonary and pharyngeal secretions
- Reduced pulmonary oedema
- Reduced peripheral oedema
- Anaesthetic effect secondary to electrolyte imbalance and production of opioid peptides
- Reduced pain through reduction in oedema around tumours and thus reduced nerve compression

Patchett (1998); NCPC (2006b); Owens (2007).

One very emotive issue involves the use of rehydration with subcutaneous or intravenous fluids (Owens 2007), as most patients stop drinking in the final days of life (Patchett 1998; NCPC 2006b). Owens (2007) points out that much of the literature on the subject is anecdotal, and there is surprisingly little research evidence on the subject. He found that the consistent theme running through the literature is that parenteral hydration causes burdensome and distressing symptoms.

Thorns and Garrard (2003) point out that it is important to distinguish between someone with an irreversible condition who is dying from their disease, and someone who is not dying but is unable to maintain their hydration and may die because of it. In the latter case, artificial hydration may be appropriate, but it is widely believed that rehydration is rarely indicated at the end of life (NCPC 2006b). The main arguments against the use of hydration are listed in Table 8.2.

It is sometimes argued that the administration of opioid analgesia is a form of passive euthanasia, but Roy (2004) maintains that one of the essential elements of dying with dignity is freedom from pain and distress that can lead to feelings of hopelessness. He argues that the proportionate use of medication in appropriate combinations and doses sufficient to relieve suffering is ethically different from the administration of medication with the intention of bringing about death.

Owens (2007) advises that all medical decisions should be made on a case-by-case basis that takes into consideration the current clinical situation, the goals of care and the potential advantages and disadvantages of any proposed treatment. Regnard and Dean (2010) provide structured guidance to assist the decision-making process, as set out in Table 8.3.

Planning care for the patient dying from lung cancer

The guidance on supportive and palliative care (NICE 2004) identified several frequently reported shortcomings in care and proposed strategies to rectify them. The identified areas of difficulty were:

Table 8.3 The ethical decision making process.

Ask:	Consider:

What courses of action are available?	• Is the patient dying or suffering from a potentially reversible condition?
	• Are there:
	  ○ Undesirable courses of action that you have discounted
	  ○ Desirable options you haven't considered
	• Is this an ethical issue or a clinical decision for which there is insufficient information to make a clear decision?
	• Ask for advice from team members or other specialists

Are you looking at the situation objectively?	• Reviewing your attitudes to issues such as age, social class, ethnicity, gender intellectual ability, lifestyle or religion. • Do you hold any prejudices?
Whose interests are being served?	Is the proposed course of action: • In the patient's best interests (and does it promote their autonomy)? • In the partner's/family's best interests? • In society's best interests? • In your/other professionals' best interests?
What values underpin this decision?	• Is the chosen course of action caring? • Is it a good use of resources? • What values are being sacrificed? • Does it involve ignoring a principle/rule you would usually comply with?
What are the consequences of your decision?	• The probable effectiveness of the proposed treatment • The suffering that may be caused • The level of awareness the individual has of his situation • Is the invasiveness of the treatment justified? Will the chosen course of action: • Benefit the client? • Cause harm to the client? • Violate anyone's rights or legitimate expectations?
Are there professional issues involved?	• Does professional guidance exist on this issue? • Are you acting within the law? • How would you justify your decision to others?

Is a course of action still unclear?	Have you:
	• Involved the patient (if they can contribute) their partner or family if they cannot?
	• Asked colleagues for their views?
	Is a course of action still unclear? How urgent is a decision?
	• If patient's deterioration is rapid use the 'rule of 3':
	  ○ If deterioration is hour by hour, wait 3 hours.
	  ○ If deterioration is day by day, wait 3 days.
	  ○ If a patient's condition deteriorates during the waiting period, this suggests that *no intervention* is required.
	  ○ If patient's condition stabilises or improves during the waiting period, further intervention *may* be appropriate.
	• If time is less urgent, consider holding a case conference or seeking legal advice

Adapted from Regnard and Dean (2010).

- Inadequate assessment of patient needs
- Poor coordination of care
- Poor face to face communication
- Lack of information
- Inadequate psychological, social and spiritual support

These failings are compounded in some areas by a lack of systems to organise and optimise palliative care in general settings and by inadequate anticipatory and discharge planning, and a range of strategies have been developed to remedy these shortcomings that together form the end of life care programme. The NHS 'End of Life Care Programme' (see http://www.endoflifecare.nhs.uk/eolc) aims to 'improve the quality of care at the end of life for all patients and enable more patients to live and die in the place of their choice' by disseminating good practice, resources and information. The programme supports the implementation of several strategies including the documents *Preferred Priorities for Care* and the *Liverpool Care Pathway for the Dying Patient*.

The *Preferred Priorities for Care* (PPC) document, formerly known as the Preferred Place of Care document (http://www.endoflifecareforadults.nhs.uk/assets/downloads/ppc_1.pdf) is a patient-held record designed to facilitate patient choice in relation to end of life care and ultimate place of death. Thus it is a form of advanced care planning that empowers the patient and promotes the discussion of difficult issues that professionals might be reluctant to explore, as well as minimizing inappropriate hospital admissions and interventions. The document can be reviewed and amended at any time as circumstances change (Pemberton *et al.* 2003).

The *Liverpool Care Pathway for the Dying Patient* (LCP) (Marie Curie Palliative Care Institute Liverpool 2009) is an integrated care pathway developed by the Specialist Palliative Care team at the Royal Liverpool University Hospital and the Marie Curie Centre in Liverpool (Kinder and Ellershaw 2003) as a vehicle for transferring the hospice model of care into other settings (Ellershaw 2003). The pathway provides a systematic, evidence-based framework for patient assessment, care planning and delivery in the last days of life, the main features of which are outlined in Table 8.4. Versions of the LCP have been developed for hospital, hospice, community and care home use, and it is permitted to make some degree of local adaptation to better reflect local practice. The tool has been widely adopted across the United Kingdom (DH 2008).

Symptom management

Griffin *et al.* (2007) identify the ten most distressing symptoms for lung cancer patients in the last 90 days of life (see Table 8.5). They explain that uncontrolled symptoms are associated in the literature with decreased health-related quality of life and shortened survival.

Detailed guidance on symptom management is beyond the remit of this chapter, but the principles of managing pain and respiratory symptoms in

Table 8.4 Features of the Liverpool Care Pathway for the Dying Patient.

Initial assessment	• Physical condition • Communication with family/other • Patient/relative or carer are aware of the impending death • Review medications – discontinue those deemed non-essential • Prescribe medication 'as required' for pain, agitation, respiratory tract secretions, nausea and vomiting and dyspnoea • Review interventions – discontinue those deemed inappropriate (e.g. blood tests, antibiotics, blood glucose monitoring, recording vital signs, oxygen, CPR status, artificial nutrition) • Psychological insight of patient/relative or carer • Communication with primary health care team/GP practice
Ongoing assessment	• Pain • Agitation • Respiratory tract secretions • Nausea • Vomiting • Breathless • Urinary problems • Bowel problems • Other symptoms • Comfort and safety regarding the administration of medication • Fluids to support individual needs • Mouthcare • Skin integrity • Personal hygiene needs • Physical environment supports individual needs • Patient's psychological well-being is maintained • Well-being of the attending relative or carer is maintained
Care after death	• Verification of death • Last offices performed according to local policy • Relative or carer understands what they need to do • Primary health care team/GP notified • Patient's death is communicated to appropriate services in the organisation

Adapted from Marie Curie Palliative Care Institute Liverpool (2009).

advanced disease will be discussed. The delivery of good end of life care requires the contribution of all members of the multidisciplinary team and meticulous attention to detail. Faull and Nyatanga (2005) highlight the essential contribution of good basic nursing care (positioning, pressure area care, mouth care, bladder and bowel care, and eye care), without which symptom control will be difficult. When the prognosis is poor, it is crucial that services respond rapidly to patient's changing needs (DH 2008).

Table 8.5 The ten most distressing symptoms for lung cancer patients in the last 90 days of life.

Symptom	%
Fatigue	93%
Decreased appetite	62%
Pain	55%
Cough	55%
Insomnia	48%
Dyspnoea	43%
Worry about the future	41%
Bowel problems	38%
Difficulty concentrating	33%
Nausea	30%

Adapted from the work of Griffin et al. (2007).

Pain

Pain is a common symptom among people with lung cancer (Griffin et al. 2007), and its prevalence is estimated to as high as 70–90% among those with advanced disease (Portenoy and Lesage 1999; Foley 2004). Pargeon and Hailey (1999) suggest that approximately 90% of people in pain could obtain adequate relief with simple drug therapies, but this is not routinely achieved in clinical practice. There is a great deal of evidence that pain is often under-treated and pain control remains inadequate (Davies and McVicar 2000; Foley 2004; Wood 2004), suggesting that little has changed since McCaffrey (1983) stated that 'pain probably disables more people than any single disease entity' (p. 1).

Uncontrolled pain has a significant, negative impact on individuals' quality of life, affecting their ability to perform activities of daily living and social and psychological functioning (Foley 2004).

According to Paz and Seymour (2004), until the 1960s pain was considered by most clinicians to be an inevitable response to tissue damage, with little recognition of the important differences between acute and chronic pain states. In addition, the physiological, psychological and sociocultural factors that contribute to our perception of pain were largely unacknowledged. Table 8.6 outlines the temporal classification of pain.

Pain assessment

Assessment is the crucial first step to managing pain, as identification of the type of pain experienced will enable us to employ the most appropriate therapeutic strategy. The adherence to a few simple principles is the key to assessment (Foley 2004). A discussion on pain can be found in Chapter 6 – the focus of this section is the management of cancer pain at the end of life.

Table 8.6 Temporal patterns of pain.

Acute pain
- Well-defined onset – follows actual injury, disease, surgery.
- Duration limited and predictable (less than 6 weeks).
- Located in area of known trauma.
- Associated with objective physical signs and hyperactivity of the autonomic nervous system (sweating, pallor, possible nausea; patient will often be unable to relax or sleep).

Chronic pain
- Persists for more than 3 months.
- Often with a less well-defined onset and no foreseeable end.
- Adaptation of the autonomic nervous system occurs, so patients lack the objective physiological signs associated with acute pain.

Breakthrough pain
- Characterised by a transient, greater than moderate, increase in pain intensity above the baseline or 'background' level experienced by the individual.
- Occurs in both acute and chronic pain states and may be due to:
  - An exacerbation of the patient's condition.
  - A voluntary or involuntary action of the patient (incident pain).
  - 'End of dose failure' – occurring towards the end of the regular analgesic dose interval.

Woodruff (1997); Foley (2004); Pasero (2006).

1. *Believe the patient's complaint of pain* (Woodruff 1997; Foley 2004). McCaffery first coined her popular definition of pain being 'whatever the patient says it is, existing whenever he says it does' in 1968 (McCaffery 1983, p. 14). While this is endlessly quoted by nurses, the literature suggests that nurses do not always believe the patient (McCaffery and Ferrell 1997; Arber 2004) and fail to acknowledge that pain is a uniquely personal experience (Bennett *et al.* 2005).

2. *Take a thorough history of the pain experience*. Be aware that patients can have more than one type of pain and that they may not all be related to the cancer or its treatment (Woodruff 1997).

As pain is an unpleasant sensory *and* emotional experience (Bennett *et al.* 2005), the history should assess all factors which may influence 'total pain' and should ask:

- When did the pain start?
- Where is it? Does it go anywhere else?
- What does it feel like?
- Is it constant or intermittent?
- Does anything exacerbate or relieve it?
- Are there any associated symptoms?
- Is the pain limiting the patient's physical or social activities?
- What does the patient think the pain is due to?

- Which analgesics have been tried and how effective were they?
- How does the pain make the patient feel? (emotional impact)
- What are the patient's fears or concerns? (psycho-social/spiritual impact)
- What is the patient's previous experience of pain and illness?

(Woodruff 1997; Foley 2004; Bennett et al. 2005).

It is also important to consider whether the patient appears to be anxious or depressed as this may greatly influence the complexity of their pain (Woodruff 1997) and affect how the individual copes with it (Foley 2004).

3. *Observe the patient's behaviour.* Some people, especially those at the end of life, may be reluctant or unable to report pain for various reasons, but the presence of pain may be evident in their behaviour. The literature identifies several non-verbal indicators of pain, including behaviours such as rapid blinking, agitation or aggression, guarding of a body part (Kaasalainen 2007), immobility, purposeless or inaccurate body movements, and protective movements including withdrawal reflex or rhythmic or rubbing movements (Feldt 2000). Facial expressions such as grimacing, wincing or frowning may also be suggestive of pain (Feldt 2000; Salmore 2002; van Herk et al. 2007).

Patients who are unable to verbalise their pain may indicate distress by using *vocal behaviours* such as crying or moaning (Kaasalainen 2007).

4. *Use a validated pain assessment tool.* These can be useful in assisting patients to communicate their subjective experience of pain (Wood 2004), and also promote continuity in the pain management process (Davies and McVicar 2000). A variety of tools are available, each with its own merits and limitations (Bird 2003; Wood 2004). These can be classified as:

- Verbal numerical scales
- Numerical rating scales
- Visual analogue scales
- Body outlines
- Pain questionnaires
- Picture scales/pain drawings (e.g. faces pain scale)
- Descriptor categories

5. *Continue to review.* Pain assessment and management is a continuous process as pain responses develop over time (Davies and McVicar 2000), and reassessment of the patient's response to treatment is essential.

Principles of cancer pain management

Bennett et al. (2005) state that approximately 30% of people with cancer do not have pain, but those who do can have four or more different types of pain. Pain may be related to:

- The tumour (70%)
- The treatment (20%)

Table 8.7 The three main types of cancer pain.

Somatic/visceral pain • Somatic pain – from skin and superficial structures • Visceral pain – from deep-seated structures	• Somatic pain is usually described as well localised, sharp, aching throbbing, or pressure like. • Visceral pain is often referred to a cutaneous site remote from the site of the lesion, and is described as diffuse, gnawing, cramping, aching, sharp or throbbing. • Usually opioid sensitive.
Bone pain	• May be poorly opioid sensitive, but usually NSAID sensitive. Radiotherapy is often beneficial.
Neuropathic pain – resulting from damage to nerve tissue	• Described variously as pins and needles, numbness, burning, shooting or stabbing. • May respond poorly or not at all to opioids – often difficult to manage and may need specialist referral for optimum management.

Wilson (2002); Klee (2004).

- Debilitating disease (<10%)
- A concurrent disorder (<10%)

(Woodruff 1997; Bennett *et al.* 2005).

Bennett *et al.* (2005) and Souhami and Tobias (2005) describe three main types of cancer-related pain (Table 8.7):

- Somatic/visceral pain – lung cancers can cause pain by direct spread into the pleural space and chest wall. Autopsies indicate an incidence of brain metastases in 65% in patients with small-cell carcinoma of the lung (Souhami and Tobias 2005).
- Bone pain – tumours of the lung frequently metastasize to the bone, particularly the vertebrae, ribs and pelvis (Souhami and Tobias 2005).
- Neuropathic pain – tumours located in the apex of the lung (Pancoast tumours) may infiltrate the brachial plexus, causing significant damage to the thoracocervical sympathetic nerve chain and the phrenic nerve or the left recurrent laryngeal nerve.

The characteristics of these are outlined in Table 8.7.

Bennett *et al.* (2005) explain that for some patients it may be possible to treat the underlying cancer and thus reduce the pain. Tumours can be shrunk by chemotherapy or radiotherapy – a single fraction of which provides good pain relief for 80% of patients with bone secondaries. However, Hanks *et al.* (2004a) explain that analgesic therapy with opioids, non-opioids and adjuvant drugs is the mainstay of cancer pain management, although other interventions may also be appropriate for many patients. Table 8.8 sets out the principles of pain management.

Table 8.8 Principles of cancer pain management.

- Selection of appropriate analgesia according to the WHO analgesic ladder
- Selection of appropriate route – orally whenever possible
- Prescription of an adequate dose
- Regular administration (*not* solely on an 'as required' basis)
- Management of breakthrough pain – 'as required' dose equivalent to the regular 4-hourly dose
- Management of any side-effects (all patients on opioids require softening and stimulating laxatives and access to an antiemetic)
- Patient/carer education
- Adjuvant therapies
- Review and reassessment of efficacy

Based on Woodruff (1997); Davies and McVicar (2000); Bennett *et al.* (2005).

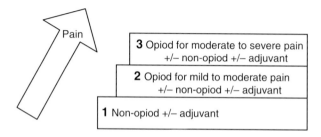

Fig. 8.1 The WHO analgesia ladder.

The World Health Organization analgesic ladder (WHO 1986, 1996) proposes a three-step approach to managing cancer pain (Fig. 8.1). As cancer pain is usually chronic, regular analgesia is required to prevent the pain recurring (NCHSPCS 1998), nevertheless, the regime should be kept as simple as possible (Woodruff 1997). If the patient's pain persists or increases, medication on the next step of the ladder is prescribed – moving always upwards and not sideways in the same efficacy group (Twycross and Wilcock 2002).

Examples of drugs used at the various steps of the analgesic ladder are outlined in Table 8.9. It is claimed that step 3 opioids are required for the majority of patients with cancer pain (NCHSPCS 1998), and that although there is now a range of agents, morphine is still considered the opioid of choice (NCHSPCS 1998; Hanks *et al.* 2004a). The recommended starting dose of morphine is 10 mg of immediate-release morphine 4 hourly (2.5–5 mg for the elderly or those with severely impaired renal or hepatic function) (NCHSPCS 1998). The opioid dose is gradually titrated upwards until the patient's pain is relieved – it should be noted that there is no maximum dose for single-agent opioid preparations when appropriately titrated (Gallagher 2007; Fudin 2008). The 'right dose' for each patient will depend on the balance between pain relief and side effects (Gallagher 2007). When good control has

Table 8.9 Classification of drugs according to the WHO analgesic ladder.

Step 1 – Non-opioids
- Paracetamol
- Aspirin
- Non-steroidal anti-inflammatory drugs (NSAIDs)

Step 2 – Opioids for mild to moderate pain
- Co-codamol 30/500
- Codeine
- Dihydrocodeine
- Dextropropoxyphene
- Tramadol

Step 3 – Opioids for moderate to severe pain
- Morphine
- Diamorphine
- Fentanyl
- Hydromorphone
- Oxycodone
- Tramadol

Pain Society (2004); Bennett *et al.* (2005); BNF (2011).

been achieved a 'sustained-release' opioid preparation may be prescribed for greater convenience and improved compliance (Forbes and Faull 1998; NHSPCS 1998). It is important that there is a strategy for the management of breakthrough pain – there should be access to a 'rescue dose' of an immediate-release opioid at a dose equivalent to the regular 4-hourly dose.

Practitioners should be cautioned that if pain remains a problem despite the opioid dose being increased, the cause of the pain should be reassessed as it may not be opioid sensitive, and seeking specialist advice should be considered (Forbes and Faull 1998). Non-opioid analgesics should be continued when opioid drugs are commenced as they have a complementary action and reduce the patient's opioid requirements (Woodruff 1997).

Managing the fears and side effects related to opioid use

There is evidence of 'professional opiophobia' (Woodruff 1997) – which results in doctors being reluctant to prescribe adequate analgesia, and nurses being reluctant to administer it if it has been prescribed on an 'as required' basis (McCaffery *et al.* 2007). This fear often leads to opioids being withheld until a patient is dying – a situation that Woodruff (1997) describes as 'archaic'. Table 8.10 considers some of the fears associated with opioid use and Table 8.11 outlines the management of possible side effects of opioids.

Bennett *et al.* (2005) recommend that the possible side effects of opioids be discussed with patients prior to commencing treatment. It is estimated that 5% of patients cannot tolerate the side effects caused by certain opioid drugs. If reducing the dose fails to remedy the situation, changing to another type of opioid may be a solution (NCHSPCS 1998).

Table 8.10 Opioids – dispelling the fears.

Addiction	When patients take opioids to combat pain, it is rare to see addiction (a psychological craving for the substance, and withdrawal symptoms when it is discontinued). Physical (but not psychological) dependence may occur if opioids are stopped suddenly.
Respiratory depression	As patients usually progress up the analgesic ladder in a controlled fashion, this is usually not a problem in clinical practice. Rather it is used to therapeutic effect in the management of breathlessness.

Melzack (1990); Hanks *et al.* (1996); Woodruff (1997); NCHSPCS (1998); Twycross and Wilcock (2001); Dickman(2003); Regnard and Hockley (2004); Bennett *et al.* (2005).

Table 8.11 Opioids – managing the side effects.

Constipation	Aperients should always be prescribed (unless contraindicated) – a softener and a stimulant.
Nausea and vomiting	Nausea may occur in 30–60% of patients, and vomiting in 10% of patients – usually temporary. Prescribe an antiemetic.
Drowsiness	Usually temporary.

NCHSPCS (1998); Bennett *et al.* (2005).

Adjuvant drugs

Adjuvant drugs is the term widely used to refer to 'co-analgesics' – those drugs that are not primarily analgesics but that have an analgesic effect in certain conditions. However, the term more correctly refers to any drug that is given with an analgesic, such as laxatives or antiemetics, given to control side effects (Lussier and Portenoy 2004). Table 8.12 outlines this group of drugs and how they can contribute to the management of pain.

Breathlessness

Unsurprisingly, respiratory symptoms are very common in patients with lung cancer, and one of most prevalent is breathlessness, affecting around 78% of people (Wade *et al.* 2005). Corner (2004) explains that breathlessness is both a disabling and a terrifying symptom, and to treat it as a purely physical problem fails to deal with the intense psychological issues involved. In recent years there has been a great deal of research into the non-pharmacological management of breathlessness (Corner *et al.* 1996; Bredin *et al.* 1999), which views the emotional experience of breathlessness as being inextricably linked

Table 8.12 The use of adjuvant drugs.

Antidepressants (e.g. amitryptyline)	Neuropathic pain
Anticonvulsants (e.g. carbamazepine, gabapentin)	Neuropathic pain
Corticosteroids (e.g dexamethasone)	Nerve compression pain
	Neuropathic pain
	Bone pain
	Painful hepatomegaly
	Raised intracranial pressure
Antispasmodics (e.g. hyoscine butylbromide)	Colicky pain

NCHSPCS (1998); Bennett *et al.* (2005).

to the sensory experience and the pathophysiological changes referred to in Chapter 6. While these strategies have been demonstrated to be beneficial, those patients who present with advanced disease or who are approaching the terminal stage of their illness are often unable to benefit significantly. Patients often fear that they will die by suffocation (Wade *et al.* 2005) and this intense dread is sometimes associated with gasping-type breathing, referred to as 'air hunger' (Regnard and Hockley 2004). Pharmacological strategies form the mainstay of management in the end stages of disease (Wade *et al.* 2005).

Oxygen therapy

Oxygen therapy is often used in hospital settings for the palliation of breathlessness, a practice that is controversial (Booth *et al.* 2004) as there is a lack of good-quality evidence to support its use (Booth *et al.* 2004; Spathis *et al.* 2006). Consequently, oxygen tends to be employed inappropriately (Wade *et al.* 2005; Spathis *et al.* 2006) and any benefit is likely to be seen in those patients who are hypoxic (Wade 2005), although even some of this group will not experience any benefit (Spathis *et al.* 2006).

However, Wade *et al.* (2005) explain that the psychological benefit of oxygen therapy is often great, and Booth *et al.* (2004) report that patients can become dependent on it and be reluctant to have it removed. Wade *et al.* (2005) suggest that this perceived benefit may come from the cooling flow of oxygen on the face, which supports the use of an electric fan to create a breeze. Booth *et al.* (2004) conclude that there is little evidence to indicate which patients are likely to benefit from oxygen therapy, and it is suggested that some form of formal assessment, such as a trial of compressed air compared with oxygen be conducted to determine its usefulness for each individual (Booth *et al.* 2004; Wade *et al.* 2005). If oxygen is indicated, it should be administered at the lowest flow rate possible to produce maximum benefit and minimal adverse effects (a rate of 2-4 L/minute is usually sufficient) (Spathis *et al.* 2006).

Wade *et al.* (2005) recommend a positive, proactive approach to the management of terminal breathlessness and suggest that someone dying with distressing breathlessness represents a failure to utilise drug therapy appropriately. They state that the combination of a parenteral opioid with a sedative anxiolytic is usually effective. Regnard and Hockley (2004) stress that the aim is not to sedate the patient but to promote relaxation and comfort.

Respiratory depressants

According to Dickman (2003) breathless patients typically experience tachypnoea and that the associated anxiety and distress can be alleviated by reducing the respiratory rate and addressing the associated anxiety.

Benzodiazepines

Wade *et al.* (2005) explain that although benzodiazepines are widely used in the management of cancer-related breathlessness, there is actually a lack of evidence to support their use. They state that any benefit gained from this group of drugs stems from their anxiolytic effect, but drowsiness, which can be disabling, is common, and there is also some evidence of ventilatory depression. Dickman (2003) and Wade *et al.* (2005) both recommend the use of benzodiazepines where anxiety is a feature in the patient's presentation. Dickman (2003) explains that lorazepam is occasionally used (0.5-1 mg sublingually), but recommends midazolam as the drug of choice in the dying patient (5-10 mg immediately or a continuous subcutaneous infusion of 10-30 mg).

Levomepromazine

Levomepromazine (a phenothiazine) may also be used to treat breathlessness associated with anxiety. Dickman (2003) suggest a starting dose of 12.5 mg daily via subcutaneous injection or infusion.

Opioids

Opioids are commonly used within specialist palliative care to palliate breathlessness - they reduce the ventilatory response to hypercapnia, hypoxia and exercise (Twycross and Wilcock 2001), reduce the respiratory rate and the level of anxiety (Dickman 2003) without significant respiratory depression (Regnard and Hockley 2004).

Twycross and Wilcock (2001) maintain that morphine reduces breathlessness by approximately 20% for up to 4 hours. For the opioid-naive patient they recommend starting with a low dose of morphine (2.5-5 mg as required) and titrate upwards according to response. If two or more doses are required in 24 hours they suggest prescribing it regularly. For the patient who is already on morphine for pain, the literature recommends increasing the 4-hourly

Table 8.13 Indications for using a continuous subcutaneous infusion (CSCI/syringe driver).

> **The oral route is not appropriate**
> - Dysphagia
> - Oral/pharyngeal lesions
> - Loss of consciousness
> - Nausea and vomiting
> - Intestinal obstruction
> - Malabsorption
> - Profound weakness
>
> **Intractable pain is NOT an indication!**

Based on Mitten (2001); Dickman (2003); Hirsch *et al.* (2005).

analgesic dose by between 25% and >100% depending on the severity of the breathlessness (Twycross and Wilcock 2001; Dickman 2003). The dose can be converted to modified-release morphine when the optimum effect is achieved. Morphine or diamorphine can also be administered via subcutaneous injection or infusion (Dickman 2003).

The last hours

As the patient moves towards the end of his or her life, the multiprofessional team should consider the appropriateness of their interventions. Inappropriate interventions would include cardiopulmonary resuscitation, blood tests, antibiotics, intravenous medication and recording vital signs (Dickman 2003). Medication should be reviewed and rationalised and non-essential medication discontinued (Marie Curie Palliative Care Institute Liverpool 2009). Glare (2003) points out that drugs originally prescribed for the management of long-term conditions or disease prevention (e.g. antibiotics, antihypertensives or statins) are largely redundant in the last days of life.

The route of drug administration should also be reviewed as towards the end of life patients frequently lapse into unconsciousness and become unable to take anything orally. Some medications can be given transdermally (e.g. fentanyl), but this should not be commenced in the terminal phase as therapeutic serum levels are not reached until 12-24 hours after application (Hanks *et al.* 2004a) and it can be difficult to establish the required dose in a rapidly changing situation (Kaye 2000). Others can be given rectally (e.g. oxycodone) – but this may be unacceptable to some people (Glare 2003). The subcutaneous route is the most convenient for the dying patient, and a continuous subcutaneous infusion (CSCI) via a syringe driver removes the need for regular injections and ensures that stable plasma levels of medication are maintained (Mitten 2001; Hanks *et al.* 2004b). Indications for the use of a CSCI are outlined in Table 8.13.

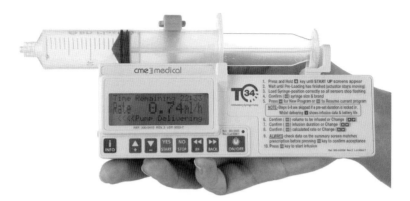

Fig. 8.2 Syringe driver used for continuous subcutaneous infusion. (Courtesy of CME McKinley, reproduced with permission.)

Possibly the most commonly used syringe drivers are the SIMS Graseby models MS16A and MS26 (Mitten 2001; Irving *et al.* 2007), although there have been a number of serious incidents involving these devices (Irving *et al.* 2007). Confusion has arisen around the fact that, in both models, the rate of administration is set in *millimetres* of fluid, based on the *length* of liquid in the syringe and *not volume*, as is usual in other infusion devices. The MS16A model administers medication at a rate set in millimetres *per hour*, and the MS26 administers medication at a rate set in millimetres *per 24 hours*. To eliminate confusion, many care providers are turning to newer devices (Irving *et al.* 2007), such as the CME McKinley T34 ambulatory syringe pump (Fig. 8.2), which administers medication at a rate set in *millilitres* per hour. It is crucial that all staff using any infusion device must have been trained and be competent in its use (Irving *et al.* 2007; British National Formulary (BNF) 2011).

Dying patients often present with some additional symptoms, such as agitation and respiratory tract secretions, and sedatives and antimuscarinics are required (Glare 2003) – Table 8.14.

While the subcutaneous route is preferred because of its convenience, many of the drugs used at the end of life are not licensed for administration by this route (Kaye 2000). Pavis and Wilcock (2001) estimate that 25% of all prescriptions in palliative medicine are for licensed drugs that are used for unlicensed indications or that are given by an unlicensed route. The Association for Palliative Medicine and the Pain Society (2001) maintain that this is a legitimate aspect of clinical practice.

Hanks *et al.* (2004b) state that a variety of drugs are often used in combination in the syringe driver, but warn that the stability and compatibility of these drugs are not known. Clinical practice in palliative care is often based on experience rather than randomised controlled studies (Higginson 1999; Kaye 2000; Jubb 2002). Hanks *et al.* (2004b) therefore advise that as few drugs as possible are combined in an infusion, ideally no more than three.

Table 8.14 Management of the common additional symptoms in the dying patient.

Agitation	• Eliminate reversible cause if possible – pain, constipation, urinary retention, opioid toxicity, hypoxia, anxiety or distress.
	• Midazolam 5–20 mg/24 hours (titrating up to 80 mg/24 hours).
	• Haloperidol 5–10 mg/24 hours.
	• Levomepromazine 12.5–100 mg/24 hours.
	• Risperidone or olanzepine may be used if the symptom persists.
Respiratory tract secretions ('the death rattle')	• Possibly more distressing to relatives than the patient – try to reassure them.
	• Positional changes to facilitate secretion drainage.
	• Glycopyrronium 0.6–1.2 mg/24 hours.
	• Hyoscine hydrobromide 1.2–2.4 mg/ 24 hours.
	• Hyoscine butylbromide 20–120 mg/ 24 hours.
	• Suction – may be very distressing for the patient.

Glare (2003); Dickman (2003); Faull and Nyatanga (2005).

Table 8.15 Drugs compatible with diamorphine.

Cyclizine	Hyoscine hydrobromide
Dexamethasone	Levomepromazine
Haloperidol	Metoclopramide
Hyoscine butylbromide	Midazolam

Adapted from BNF (2011).

Dickman (2003) maintains that no more than this is needed to mange most symptoms at the end of life - usually an analgesic, an antiemetic/sedative and an antimuscarinic.

Diamorphine is the opioid most commonly used in a CSCI owing to its solubility (Dickman 2003; Hirsch *et al*. 2005), and the literature maintains that it is compatible with the drugs indicated in Table 8.15.

The compatibility of drugs is dependent on several factors, such as the nature of the drugs being mixed, the diluent used and the concentration of the drug (Hanks *et al*. 2004b). Most centres use water for injection as the diluent in CSCIs as the use of sodium chloride 0.9% increases the likelihood of precipitation when more than one drug is used (Hirsch *et al*. 2005; BNF 2011).

Table 8.16 Critical nursing behaviours.

Responding during the death scene	● Maintaining a sense of calm
	● Maintaining family involvement
Providing comfort	● Reducing physical discomfort (especially pain)
Responding to anger	● Showing respect and empathy even when anger is directed at the nurse
Enhancing the quality of life of the patient and family	● Helping patients to do what is important to them
Responding to the family	● Responding to the family's need for information
	● Behaviours that reduce the potential for future regret
	● Behaviours that involve the family in patient care as much as they wish

Adapted from Degner *et al.* (1991).

For example, cyclizine may precipitate at concentrations above 10 mg/mL *or* if mixed with sodium chloride 0.9% *or* as the concentration of diamorphine relative to cyclizine increases (BNF 2011).

Social care

Spichiger (2008) found that, while patients and their families expect clinical competence from health care professionals, what they particularly valued was 'friendliness, cheerfulness and good manners ... grounded in empathy consideration and respect' (p. 229).

Degner *et al.* (1991) identify several behaviours demonstrated by nurses delivering end of life care that were considered positive (Table 8.16).

Royak-Schaler *et al.* (2006) found that satisfaction with end of life care was closely related to the perceived quality of communication that patients and family members had with the health care team. The Liverpool Care Pathway, requires professionals to explore the patients' and their families' awareness of the situation, and ensure that they have the opportunity to discuss those issues that are important to them (Marie Curie Palliative Care Institute Liverpool 2009).

Heming and Colmer (2003) explain that we live in a diverse multicultural and multifaith community and it is important that patients' and families' spiritual and religious needs are catered for. For some this may involve a chaplain or minister to meet a particular religious need such as prayer or ritual, whereas for others it might be someone sitting quietly with the person or listening to their concerns (Speck 2003). For those cultural groups who have more expressive forms of mourning, a side room might be needed to meet their needs (Wilkinson and Mula 2003).

Table 8.17 Factors that help those anticipating or experiencing a loss.

Show genuine concern and caring	Do not avoid them because you feel uncomfortable/embarrassed/helpless
Be available to listen and help with whatever they need	Avoid platitudes – e.g. 'I know how you feel', *or* suggesting they should be grateful for the loss *or* finding something positive about their loss - e.g. 'it's a happy release for X'
Say you are sorry for the death and for their pain	Avoid telling them what they should do or how they should feel
Allow expression of feelings	Do not avoid mentioning the loss for fear of upsetting them/reminding them of their pain
Encourage them to be patient with themselves	Do not judge their emotions – e.g. you shouldn't feel like that'
Allow them to talk about their loss as much as they wish	Avoid blocking the discussion
Reassure them that they did all they could	Avoid saying anything that might suggest that the loss was their fault

Adapted from Wilkinson and Mula (2003).

Heming and Colmer (2003) explain that families can begin preparing for an expected loss weeks or months before the patient actually dies and will need a great deal of support during this time. Wilkinson and Mula (2003) outline those behaviours that are helpful to those who are facing bereavement or have recently been bereaved (Table 8.17).

Summary

While the provision of end of life care is often challenging, it is always rewarding (Heming and Colmer 2003). The way in which loved ones are cared for in their last hours makes a lasting impression in the memories of relatives (DH 2008).

The Department of Health (DH 2008) points to the fact that the way in which the dying are cared for is an indicator of how society cares for the sick and vulnerable, and that end of life care should be regarded as a core activity of all who work in health and social care. Faull (1998) expands on this view, stating that palliative care is an integral part of total patient management, regardless of the actual care setting.

Saunders in 1958 outlined the scale of the challenge that health care professionals face in trying to provide the confidence and security sought by dying patients and their families, stressing that 'understanding and prompt dealing with their ills and anxieties as they occur is of more real value than false optimism' (see Saunders 2006, p. 10).

Spichiger (2008) argues that professionals can significantly improve the experience of patients and their families at the end of life by 'humanising the hospital setting', by recognising them as individuals, and by enabling them to continue and complete their lives as they wish. Griffin *et al.* (2003) make a series of recommendations to improve end of life care for people with lung cancer and thus reach the standard set by Dame Cicely Saunders, the founder of the modern hospice movement 50 years ago. These include:

- An increased focus on the patient's experience of illness – with professionals demonstrating increased levels of empathy, sensitivity and compassion.
- Patients should be informed of the diagnosis and its meaning, and be invited to participate in discussions about appropriate goals of treatment.
- Early involvement of specialist palliative care services.
- Access for staff to communication skills training.

The essence of good end of life care for patients with lung cancer encapsulates a holistic approach as summed up by the founder of the modern hospice movement who pioneered research into symptom management:

> You matter because you are you, and you matter until the last moment of your life. We will do all that we can to help you not only to die peacefully, but to live until you die'
>
> Dame Cicely Saunders, cited in Faull (1998, p. 2)

References

Arber, A. (2004) Is pain what the patient says it is? Interpreting an account of pain. *International Journal of Palliative Nursing*, **10** (10), 491–496.

Ariès, P. (1993) Death denied. In: *Death, Dying and Bereavement* (eds D. Dickenson and M. Johnson), pp. 11–15. SAGE Publications and Open University, London.

Association for Palliative Medicine and the Pain Society (2001) *The Use of Drugs Beyond Licence in Palliative Care and Pain Management: A Position Statement* [on-line]. Available at: http://www.palliative-medicine.org/resources/images/Drugs_doc.pdf. Accessed 18 July 2011.

Bennett, M., Forbes, K. and Faull, C. (2005) The principles of pain management. In: *Handbook of Palliative Care* (eds C. Faull, Y. Carter, and L. Daniels), 2nd edn, pp. 116–149. Blackwell, Oxford.

Bird, J. (2003) Selection of pain measurement tools. *Nursing Standard*, **18** (13), 33–39.

Booth, S., Anderson, H., Swannick, M., Wade, R., Kite, S. and Johnson, M. (2004) The use of oxygen in the palliation of breathlessness. A report of the expert working group of the scientific committee of the association of palliative medicine. *Respiratory Medicine*, **98**, 66–77.

Bredin, M., Corner, J., Krishnasamy, M., Plant, H., Bailey, C. and A'Hern, R. (1999) Multicentre randomised controlled trial of nursing intervention for breathlessness in patients with lung cancer. *British Medical Journal*, **318**, 901–904.

Brent, S.B., Speece, M.W., Gates, M.F., Mood, D. and Kaul, M. (1991) The contribution of death-related experiences to health care providers' attitudes toward dying patients: I. Graduate and undergraduate nursing students. *Omega: Journal of Death and Dying*, **23**, 249-278.

BNF (2011) *British National Formulary 61* [on-line]. Available at: http://bnf.org/bnf/bnf/current/128644.htm. Accessed 18 July 2011.

Cancer Research UK (2011) *Latest UK Cancer Incidence (2008) and Mortality (2008) Summary June 2011* [on-line]. Available at: http://info.cancerresearchuk.org/prod_consump/groups/cr_common/@nre/@sta/documents/generalcontent/cr_072109.pdf. Accessed 18 July 2011.

Clark, D. (1993) Death in staithes. In: *Death, Dying and Bereavement* (eds D. Dickenson and M. Johnson), pp. 4-10. The Open University and SAGE Publications, London.

Corner, J. (1993) The impact of nurses' encounters with cancer on their attitudes towards the disease. *Journal of Advanced Nursing*, **2**, 363-372.

Corner, J. (2004) Working with difficult symptoms. In: *Palliative Care Nursing: Principles and Evidence for Practice* (eds S. Payne, J. Seymour and C. Ingleton), pp. 241-259. Open University Press, Buckingham.

Corner, J., Plant, H., A'Hern, R. and Bailey, C. (1996) Non-pharmacological intervention for breathlessness in lung cancer. *Palliative Medicine*, **10**, 299-305.

Davies, J. and McVicar, A. (2000) Issues in pain control 1: assessment and education. *International Journal of Palliative Nursing*, **6**(2), 58-65.

Degner, L.F., Gow, C.M. and Thompson, L.A. (1991) Critical nursing behaviors in care for the dying. *Cancer Nursing*, **14** (5), 246-253.

DH (2000) *The NHS Cancer Plan*. Department of Health, London.

DH (2008) *End of Life Care Strategy - promoting high quality care for all adults at the end of life*. Department of Health, London.

Dickman, A. (2003) Section 2 of Symptom control in care of the dying. In: *Care of the Dying - A Pathway to Excellence* (eds J. Ellershaw and S. Wilkinson), pp. 48-55. Oxford University Press, Oxford.

Ellershaw, J. (2003) Introduction. In: *Care of the Dying - A Pathway to Excellence* (eds J. Ellershaw and S. Wilkinson), pp. xi-xii. Oxford University Press, Oxford.

Ellershaw, J. (2011) Introduction. In: *Care of the Dying - A Pathway to Excellence* (eds J. Ellershaw and S. Wilkinson), 2nd edn, pp. xix-xxii. Oxford University Press, Oxford.

Ellershaw, J. and Murphy, D. (2011) What is the Liverpool Care Pathway for the Dying Patient (LCP)?. In: *Care of the Dying - A Pathway to Excellence* (eds J. Ellershaw and S. Wilkinson), 2nd edn, pp. 15-31. Oxford University Press, Oxford.

Ellershaw, J. and Ward, C. (2003). Care of the dying patient: the last hours or days of life. *British Medical Journal*, **326**, 30-34.

Faull, C. (1998) The history and principles of palliative care. In: *Handbook of Palliative Care* (eds C. Faull, Y. Carter, and R. Woof), pp. 1-12. Blackwell Science, Oxford.

Faull, C. and Nyatanga, B. (2005) Terminal care and dying. In: *Handbook of Palliative Care* (eds C. Faull, Y. Carter, and L. Daniels), 2nd edn, pp. 380-408. Blackwell, Oxford.

Feldt, K.S. (2000) The checklist of nonverbal pain indicators (CNPI). *Pain Management Nursing*, **1** (1), 13-21.

Foley, K.M. (2004) Acute and chronic cancer pain syndromes. In: *Oxford Textbook of Palliative Medicine* (eds D. Doyle, G. Hanks, N.I. Cherny and K. Calman), 3rd ed, pp. 298-316. Oxford University Press, Oxford.

Forbes, K. and Faull, C. (1998) The principles of pain management. In: *Handbook of Palliative Care* (eds C. Faull, Y. Carter, and R. Woof), pp. 99-133. Blackwell Science, Oxford.

Frommelt, C.H. (1991) The effects of death education on nurses' attitudes toward caring for terminally ill persons and their families. *American Journal of Hospice and Palliative Care*, **8** (5): 37-43.

Fudin, J. (2008) What is the maximum safe dose of opioids? Available at http://www.medscape.com/viewarticle/569913. Accessed 18 July 2011.

Gallagher, R. (2007) Multiple opioids in pain management. *Canadian Family Physician*, **53**, 2119-2120.

Glare, P. (2003) Section 1 of Symptom control in care of the dying. In: *Care of the Dying - A Pathway to Excellence* (eds J. Ellershaw and S. Wilkinson), pp. 42-48. Oxford University Press, Oxford.

Griffin, J.P., Nelson, J.E., Koch, K.A., *et al.* (2003) End-of-life care in patients with lung cancer. *Chest*, **123**, 312S-331S.

Griffin, J.P., Loch, K.A., Nelson, J.E. and Cooley, M.E. (2007) Palliative care consultation, quality-of-life measurements, and bereavement for end-of-life care in patients with lung cancer - AACP evidence-based clinical practice guidelines (2nd edition). *Chest*, **132**, 404S-422S.

Hanks, G., Cherny, N.I. and Fallon, M. (2004a) Opioid analgesic therapy. In: *Oxford Textbook of Palliative Medicine* (eds D. Doyle, G. Hanks, N.I. Cherny and K. Calman), 3rd ed, pp. 316-341. Oxford University Press, Oxford.

Hanks, G., Roberts, C.J.C. and Davies, A.N. (2004b) Principles of drug use in palliative medicine. In: *Oxford Textbook of Palliative Medicine* (eds D. Doyle, G. Hanks, N.I. Cherny and K. Calman), 3rd ed, pp. 213-225. Oxford University Press, Oxford.

Hanks, G.W., de Conno, F., Ripamonti, C., (1996) Morphine in cancer pain: modes of administration. *British Medical Journal*, **312**, 823-826.

Hanson, E. (2004) Supporting families of terminally ill persons. *Palliative Care Nursing: Principles and Evidence for Practice* (eds S. Payne, J. Seymour and C. Ingleton), pp. 329-350. Open University Press, Buckingham.

Healthcare Commission (2007) *Spotlight on Complaints - a Report on Second Stage Complaints about the NHS in England*. Commission for Healthcare Audit and Inspection, London.

Heming, D. and Colmer, A. (2003) Care of dying patients. *Nursing Standard*, **19** (18), 47-54.

Higginson, I. (1999) Evidence based palliative care. *British Medical Journal*, **319**, 462-463.

Hirsch, C., Johnson, J. and Faull, C. (2005) Medicines management in palliative care. In: *Handbook of Palliative Care* (eds C. Faull, Y. Carter, and L. Daniels), 2nd edn, pp. 409-436. Blackwell, Oxford.

Irvine, B. (1993) Teaching palliative nursing to students. *Nursing Standard*, **7** (50), 37-39.

Irving, M.J., Irving, R.J. and Sutherland, S. (2007) Graseby MS16A and MS26 syringe drivers: reported effectiveness of an online learning programme. *International Journal of Palliative Nursing*, **13** (2), 56-61.

Jubb, A.M. (2002) Palliative care research: trading ethics for an evidence base. *Journal of Medical Ethics*, **28** (6), 342-346.

Kaasalainen, S. (2007) Pain assessment in older adults with dementia. *Journal of Gerontological Nursing*, (June), 6-10.

Kaye, P. (2000) *Flow-Charts for Symptom Control*. EPL Publications, Northampton.

Kinder, C. and Ellershaw, J. (2003) How to use the Liverpool Care Pathway for the Dying Patient? In: *Care of the Dying - A Pathway to Excellence* (eds J. Ellershaw and S. Wilkinson), pp. 11-41. Oxford University Press, Oxford.

Klee, M. (2004) *The Puzzle of Pain* [on-line]. *Available* at: http://www.symptomcontrol.info/110.0.html. Accessed 21 July 2011.

Kubler-Ross, E. (1970) *On Death and Dying*. Tavistock Publications, London.

Lanceley, A. (2008) The impact of cancer on health care professionals. In: *Cancer Nursing: Care in Context* (eds J. Corner and C. Bailey), 2nd edn, pp. 153-171. Blackwell, Oxford.

Lussier, D. and Portenoy, R.K. (2004) Adjuvant analgesics in pain management. In: *Oxford Textbook of Palliative Medicine* (eds D. Doyle, G. Hanks, N.I. Cherny and K. Calman), 3rd ed, pp. 349-378. Oxford University Press, Oxford.

Marie Curie Palliative Care Institute Liverpool (2009). *The Liverpool Care of the Dying Pathway (LCP) Core Documentation*. (version 12). Avaialbale at http://www.mcpcil.org.uk/liverpool-care-pathway/Updated%20LCP%20pdfs/LCP_V12_Core_Documentation_FINAL_%28Example%29.pdf. Accessed 17th February 2011.

Melzack, R. (1990) The tragedy of needless pain. *Scientific American*, **262** (2), 19-25.

McCaffrey, M. (1983) *Nursing the Patient in Pain*. Harper and Rowe, London.

McCaffrey, M. and Ferrell, B. (1997) Nurses' knowledge of pain assessment and management: how much progress have we made? *Journal of Pain and Symptom Management*, **14** (3), 175-188.

McCaffrey, M., Pasero, C. and Ferrell, B.R. (2007) Nurses' decisions about opioid doses. *American Journal of Nursing*, **107** (12), 35-39.

McCaughan, E. and Parahoo, K. (2000) Attitudes to cancer of medical and surgical nurses in a district general hospital. *European Journal of Oncology Nursing*, **4** (3), 162-170.

Mitten, T. (2001) Subcutaneous drug infusions: a review of problems and solutions. *International Journal of Palliative Nursing*, **7** (2), 75-85.

NCHSPCS (1998) *Guidelines for Managing Cancer Pain in Adults*. London: National Council for Specialist Palliative Care Services.

NCPC (2006a) *End of Life Care Strategy*. National Council for Palliative Care, London.

NCPC (2006b) *Changing Gear: Guidelines for Managing the Last days of Life in Adults*. National Council for Palliative Care, London.

National Statistics (2007) *News Release: Cancer Survival Increases in England*. National Statistics, London.

NHS End of Life Care Programme. Available at: [on-line] http://www.endoflifecareforadults.nhs.uk/. Accessed 18 July 2011.

NHS End of Life Care Programme - Preferred Priorities for Care (PPC). Available at: http://www.endoflifecareforadults.nhs.uk/tools/core-tools/preferredpriorities forcare. Accessed 18 July 2011.

NHS Executive (1998) *Improving Outcomes in Lung Cancer*. Department of Health, London.

NICE (2004) *Improving Supportive and Palliative Care for Adults with Cancer*. National Institute for Clinical Excellence, London.

Owens, D.A. (2007) Hydration in the terminally ill: a review of the literature. *Journal of Hospice and Palliative Nursing*, **9** (3), 122-123.

Pain Society (2004) *Recommendations for the Appropriate Use of Opioids for Persistent Non-Cancer Pain*. The Pain Society, London.

Pargeon, K.L. and Hailey, B.J. (1999) Barriers to effective pain management. *Journal of Pain and Symptom Management*, **18** (5), 358-368.

Pasero, C. (2006) Management of breakthrough pain in the cancer patient. *US Oncological Disease* [on-line]. Available at http://www.touchbriefings.com/pdf/2460/pasero.pdf. Accessed 18 July 2011.

Patchett, M. (1998) Providing hydration for the terminally ill patient. *International Journal of Palliative Nursing*, **4** (3), 143-146.

Pavis, H. and Wilcock, A. (2001) Prescribing of drugs for use outside their licence in palliative care: survey of specialists in the United Kingdom. *British Medical Journal*, **323**, 484-485.

Paz, S. and Seymour, J. (2004) Pain – theories, evaluation and management. In: *Palliative Care Nursing: Principles and Evidence for Practice* (eds S. Payne, J. Seymour and C. Ingleton), pp. 260-298. Open University Press, Buckingham.

Pemberton, C., Storey, L. and Howard, A. (2003) The preferred place of care document: an opportunity for communication. *International Journal of Palliative Nursing*, **9** (10), 439-441.

Pennell, M. and Corner, J. (2001) Palliative care and cancer. In: *Cancer Nursing: Care in Context* (eds J. Corner and C. Bailey), pp. 517-534. Blackwell Science, Oxford.

Portenoy, R.K. and Lesage, P. (1999) The management of cancer pain. *The Lancet*, **353** (9165), 1695-1700.

Regnard, C. and Dean, M. (2010) *A Guide to Symptom Relief in Palliative Care*, 5th edn. Radcliffe Publishing, Oxford.

Regnard, C. and Hockley, J. (2004) *A Guide to Symptom Relief in Palliative Care*, 5th edn. Radcliffe Medical Press, Oxford.

Roy, D.J. (2004) Euthanasia and withholding treatment. In: *Oxford Textbook of Palliative Medicine* (eds D. Doyle, G. Hanks, N.I. Cherny and K. Calman), 3rd ed, pp. 84-97. Oxford University Press, Oxford.

Royak-Schaler, R., Gadalla, S.M., Lemkau, J.P., Ross, D.D., Alexander, C. and Scott, D. (2006) family perspectives on communication with healthcare providers during end-of-life cancer care. *Oncology Nursing Forum*, **33** (6), 753-760.

Sacred Congregation for the Doctrine of the Faith (1980) *Declaration on Euthanasia*. Catholic Truth Society, London.

Salmore, R. (2002) Development of a new pain scale: Colorado behavioural numerical pain scale for sedated adult patients undergoing gastrointestinal procedures. *Gastroenterology Nursing*, **25** (6), 257-262.

Saunders, C. (1958) Dying of cancer. In: Saunders, C. (2006) *Cicely Saunders – Selected Writings 1958 – 2004*. Oxford University Press, Oxfords, pp. 1-11.

Seymour, J. and Ingleton, C. (2004) Overview. In: *Palliative Care Nursing: Principles and Evidence for Practice* (eds S. Payne, J. Seymour and C. Ingleton), pp. 15-38.

Singleton, J. and McLaren, S. (1995) *Ethical Foundations of Health Care – Responsibilities in Decision Making*. Mosby, London.

Souhami, R. and Tobias, J. (2005) *Cancer and Its Management*. 5th edn. Blackwell, Oxford.

Spathis, A., Wade, R. and Booth, S. (2006) Oxygen in the palliation of breathlessness. In: *Dyspnoea in Advanced Disease* (eds S. Booth and D. Dudgeon). Oxford University Press.

Speck, P. (2003) Spiritual/religious issues in care of the dying. In: *Care of the Dying – A Pathway to Excellence* (eds J. Ellershaw and S. Wilkinson), pp. 90-105. Oxford University Press, Oxford.

Spichiger, E. (2008) Living with terminal illness: patient and family experiences of hospital end-of-life care. *International Journal of Palliative Nursing*, **14** (5), 220-228.

Thompson, I.E., Melia, K.M., Boyd, K.M. and Horsburgh, D. (2006) *Nursing Ethics*, 5th edn. Churchill Livingstone Elsevier, Edinburgh.

Thorns, A. and Garrard, E. (2003) Ethical issues in care of the dying. In: *Care of the Dying – A Pathway to Excellence* (eds J. Ellershaw and S. Wilkinson), pp. 62-73. Oxford University Press, Oxford.

Twycross, R. and Wilcock, A. (2001) *Symptom Management in Advanced Cancer*, 3rd edn. Radcliffe Medical Press, Oxford.

van Herk, R., van Dijk, M., Baar, F.P.M., Tibboel, D. and de Wit, R. (2007) Observation scales for pain assessment in older adults with cognitive impairments or communication difficulties. *Nursing Research*, **56** (1), 34-43.

Wade, R., Booth, S. and Wilcock, A. (2005) The management of respiratory symptoms. In: *Handbook of Palliative Care* (eds C. Faull, Y. Carter, and L. Daniels), 2nd edn, pp. 185-207. Blackwell, Oxford.

WHO (1986) *Cancer Pain Relief*. World Health Organization, Geneva.

WHO (1996) *Cancer Pain Relief*. World Health Organization, Geneva.

WHO (2002) *National Cancer Control Programmes. Policies and Managerial Guidelines*, 2nd edn. World Health Organization, Geneva.

Wilkinson, S. (1997) Does education assist cancer nurses with their fear of death? *European Journal of Cancer*, **33** (1008), 308.

Wilkinson, S. and Mula, C. (2003) Communication in the care of the dying. In: *Care of the Dying - A Pathway to Excellence* (eds J. Ellershaw and S. Wilkinson), pp. 74-89. Oxford University Press, Oxford.

Wilson, M. (2002) Overcoming the challenges of neuropathic pain. *Nursing Standard*, **16** (33), 47-53.

Winslow, M. and Clark, D. (2005) *St Joseph's Hospice, Hackney - A Century of Caring in the East End of London*. Observatory Publications, Lancaster.

Wood, S. (2004) Factors influencing the selection of appropriate pain assessment tools. *Nursing Times*, **100** (35), 42-47.

Woodruff, R. (1997) *Cancer Pain*. Asperula, Melbourne.

Chapter 9

Quality of Life in Lung Cancer

Alison Leary

Key points

- Quality of life has defied definition.
- Quality of life is personal and subjective.
- Health-related quality of life instruments can be used to gain some insight into quality of life in patients with cancer.
- Holistic assessment and meeting the needs of patients and families with cancer are central to good quality of life.

Introduction

Quality of life has defied objective definition for centuries; scholars such as Cicero (Cicero trans. Grant 1971) comment on what they considered 'the good life'. Despite this, the term is often used by both patient and clinicians as a preferred outcome to treatment and, having value, it is very subjective and personal.

A search of the medical databases of the last forty years (1970 to writing) yields much in terms of literature with respect to lung cancer and to quality of life, but little combining the two areas, particularly outside the context of randomised clinical trials examining quality of life as an end point of a drug trial. Definitions of quality of life range vastly from the holistic World Health Organization definition (WHO 1993) through social and physical well-being of patients to the ability to lead a fulfilling life (Bullinger *et al.* 1993). Nursing and other health-related literature yields the majority of quality of life references (Koller and Lorentz 2002) but there is little given in the way of definition of the term. Quality of life has until recently been viewed as a constant (Carr *et al.* 2001).

Lung Cancer: A Multidisciplinary Approach, First Edition. Edited by Alison Leary.
© 2012 Blackwell Publishing Ltd. Published 2012 by Blackwell Publishing Ltd.

Cancer: the journey, the individual and society

There is an abundance of clinical trial literature examining health-related or functional quality of life in lung cancer trials. These tend to be based around functional ability such as activities of daily living. The experience of the lung cancer journey, including treatment, is something rarely examined. Cancer care and treatment cannot take place in a vacuum as individuals who experience disease are still individuals. This is expressed eloquently by Harvey Cushing:

> A physician is obligated to consider more than the diseased organ, more even than the whole man – he must view the man within his world.
> Harvey Cushing 1869–1939 (Faull and Woof 2002)

There is much published work on cancer and its meaning. A study by Krishnasamy and Wilkie in 1999 (prior to launch of the NHS Cancer Plan in 2000) examined the needs of lung cancer patients and their carers and professionals' perceptions of such needs. This study remains one of very few that looks at these issues in any depth. There are many possible reasons for this: the possibility of nihilism in the treatment of lung cancer or the comparative funding issues (Roy Castle Foundation, personal communication, 2009). The cancer reform and modernisation work of the last 10 years has meant a more streamlined and confluent approach to care, particularly around the area of first presentation from primary care and into secondary or tertiary referral where many bottlenecks to patient movement had been identified. The implementation of the modernisation agenda means that the cancer journey is now much faster, with an initial target of diagnosis to definitive treatment of 31 days in 2001 (Department of Health (DH) 2000a) and currently a target of GP presentation to definitive treatment of 62 days (DH 2003). In a time of uncertainty this allows little time for the adaptation process, which can cause increased psychological pain (Houldin 2000). The 'patient journey' along with the organisation of care for people with cancer can therefore become a much more negative experience than it already is (DH 2000a).

Another significant area of change in the management of the cancer pathway is the much earlier (often pre-diagnosis) involvement of other health care professionals such as clinical nurse specialists and oncologists. Cancer care is now managed by teams rather than, for example, an individual surgeon or physician as was often the norm (Cancer Services Collaborative 2001). Patients value having a contactable key professional at all stages of the journey (Krishnasamy and Wilkie 1999; Schou and Hewison 1999; DH 2000b, 2007) and the multiprofessional team has made this a realistic possibility in practice.

Technological developments such as general anaesthesia and microscopy have allowed science and medicine to define cancer. By the early twentieth century, cancer became a disease state in it own right. Owing to the limited availability of analgesia and the fact that surgery was not as technically advanced, the person with a tumour would typically have more visible symptoms. Non-healing, fungating wounds, poorly controlled pain and debilitation would have been visible to those around the person. The fact that some of these visible signs may have been similar to those of syphilis may have contributed to the common belief that cancer was contagious (Holland 1998).

This may account for the stigma that is attached to cancer today and the stigmatising effect that Scambler has defined as 'a condition which sets apart the possessor from "normal" people' (Scambler 1991). It is something of an axiom now that cancer is a stigmatising illness. Scambler's classic work goes on to describe the perceived exclusion of those with rectal cancer as a result of labelling (Scambler 1991). The person becomes the person with cancer despite the previous role they held in society and may still hold. Repeated studies have shown this (Mathiesen and Stam 1995).

The epidemiology of lung cancer and the link with smoking have already been discussed in Chapter 1, but this link is almost ingrained into society and lay belief as a result of many health education initiatives. Tobacco use is recognised as a risk factor in lung cancer, but there is limited information about how a smoking history impacts on the emotional distress of those diagnosed with lung cancer. There have been some studies that examine causal attribution of lung cancer in populations who smoke or have used tobacco in the past. These have shown that past tobacco use correlates with greater emotional distress (Berckman and Austin 1993). It is also thought that anger and resentment may be exhibited by those who have no smoking history themselves but who may have been exposed to second-hand smoke at home or work (Sarna et al. 1993). The study by Chapple et al. (2004) reports that participants (adults with lung cancer) felt stigmatised to the point at which they felt the interactions with family, friends and doctors was often affected, with some participants concealing their disease. This occurred in smokers and non-smokers (Chapple et al. 2004).

In addition, in terms of Parsons' classic work on 'the sick role' (Parsons 1951), a person with advanced lung cancer cannot realistically be expected to fulfil the obligations of recovery and for the person with advanced lung cancer it is unlikely to be temporary state. The person with advanced lung cancer may also wish to fulfil the obligation of cooperation with medical practice. This is likely to be chemotherapy, which offers only a limited survival benefit. Should persons with advanced lung cancer be exempted from these obligations? Would this obligation extend to prioritising quality of life above other medical treatment?

The person who has cancer as a pathological disease state will also experience the psychosocial dimension of 'having cancer'. Suffering is inherent in cancer, as discussed in Chapter 7 and the alleviation of suffering is a precursor to quality of life. One way to alleviate the social isolation of cancer that causes suffering is by social ties. The benefits of having social ties (and as a corollary, the lack of social ties) are illustrated by the model of pathways linking the social environment to cancer (Helgeson et al. 1998). This relationship and its proposed effect are shown in Figure 9.1.

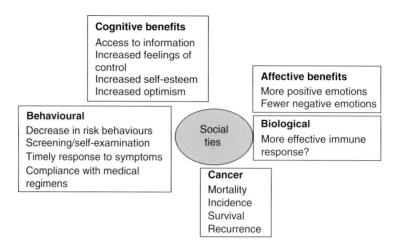

Fig. 9.1 The benefits of social ties.

Doing the work of cancer and quality of life

Apart from the physical effects of disease and side effects from treatment such as chemotherapy and radiotherapy, the majority of work that has to be done by patients with cancer is around managing the treatment calendar (appointments with key professionals, investigations, infringement into everyday life) (Schou and Hewison 1999). Easier negotiation of the calendar or 'cancer trajectory' by standardisation was one of the motivations of initiatives such as the modernisation agenda and the Cancer Plan (DH 2000a). Despite much success in smoothing this pathway, the complexity of the work appears to remain (DH 2007). Many clinicians in practice will appreciate that the cancer trajectory is not always a straight line and this causes more work for patients, physically, organisationally or in terms of emotional labour. Many patients negotiate the calendar by accessing the key professional who has power or influence over the calendar (Schou and Hewison 1999; Leary and Corrigan 2005). This role has now been recognised and supported, usually by means of clinical nurse specialists (DH 2007) and the recognition of the Key Worker role (NICE 2005). It is now recognised that although medical care can reduce the impact of illness, inattentive care can increase the impact of disruption and therefore become a source of suffering (Cassell 2004).

Towards an understanding of the meaning of quality of life in lung cancer

Survival rates and side effects have become the dominant constructs of cancer treatment and cancer care, to the detriment of more supportive and patient focused approaches. The concept of quality of life introduced to address this has failed to temper the language of oncology.

> Professor Jessica Corner, The Robert Tiffany Lecture 1996,
> 9th International Conference on Cancer Nursing

Even with the onset of cancer modernisation, quality of life in cancer remains resolutely functional. The quote above from Jessica Corner still resonates: despite great progress in cancer modernisation, living well with and beyond cancer has only more recently become in focus (DH 2007).

Quality of life scoring and assessment are based around carefully constructed questionnaires designed to measure the impact of health-related quality of life in patients taking part in clinical trials. Such measures are useful comparators, but do they 'measure' quality of life?

> Scientists may use rating scales and visual analogue scales to measure pain and they may even invent scoring systems quantifying types of handicap, but when they talk about measuring quality of life they have gone too far.
>
> Henrik Wulff (Wulff 1999)

The statement of Wulff (1999) above was cited in a review and deconstruction of the concept of quality of life (Koller and Lorenz 2002) that demonstrates not only the difficulty of developing such a definition but also the apparent scepticism about the value of doing so.

Quality of life is apparent in two contexts: authors seek either to define quality of life or to measure quality of life. This may seem a logical path to take, but it means that the literature lacks integration. For example, this fragmentation makes it difficult for a clinician to introduce quality of life assessment into practice without in-depth exploration of the two areas, unless a formulaic approach is used. This is exactly the situation at present and explains the dominance of questionnaires and quality-of -life tools in practice, particularly in the context of health economics. The definition from the Oxford English Dictionary (1995) of quality of life as '... a vague and ethereal entity' serves to illustrate the difficulty in attempting to define quality of life and illustrates the difficulty also faced by the researcher in this area in trying to find that definition. When quality of life has been discussed in the literature, it has usually been in terms that vary widely from the 'need-based' theories of authors such as Maslow (Maslow 1954) to expressions of the value or excellence of life and the word 'quality' being used in an evaluative sense (Meeberg 1993). Scholars argue that this is such an enormous area of study that it is almost impossible to define quality of life (Stegbaur 1994). This was also true in application of the term quality of life.

Quality of life is a multilevel concept reflecting macrosocietal and sociodemographic influences and also the micro concerns of individuals' experiences, circumstances, health, social well-being, values, perceptions and psychology (Bowling et al. 2003). Quality of life became a focus for nursing practice in the

1980s and, as more definitions emerged, the concept receded (Mast 1995). It is possible that as nursing has evolved with such rapidity, many terms have become ambiguous. Quality of life is of particular interest to nurses and nurse researchers because much value is placed on the evaluation of nursing interventions and quality of life could be perceived as an outcome measure. This is demonstrated by the liberal use of the term 'quality of life' in the nursing literature. The Oncology Nursing Society, for example, cited 'quality of life' as among its top three priorities, without definition (Stetz et al. 1995).

Incidence, survival and mortality have historically been used to map cancer pathology and success of treatment (Fraumen et al. 1993) and this is reflected in Corner's assertion above (Corner 1997). The oncology literature is dominated by studies in which 5-year survival, prognosis and tumour response are the main themes. This is not surprising, but as the primary language of cancer they reflect the fear of the disease and support the association of cancer with death. The introduction of quality of life and health-related quality of life has not tempered this language; however, the criticism of the over-emphasis on survival as the sole legitimate aim of treatment has led to greater consideration of factors such as quality of life (Corner 1997).

Oncology was one of the first areas of medicine to include the assessment of the impact of treatment on functioning as part of the treatment agenda. The work of Karnofsky and colleagues is an example of this (Karnofsky et al. 1948; Schou and Hewison 1999). In general terms, cancer is difficult to cure and most types of treatment induce some kind of toxicity. In the late 1970s and early 1980s, consideration of quality of life began to emerge in the oncology literature. Some authors have attributed this to technological progress and the increasingly complex treatment options that became available (de Haes and van Knippenberg 1985). Generally, quality of life in oncology is operationalised as functional status, so there has been a strong argument that quality of life in oncology essentially still has a biomedical focus through a dependence on a 'functional living' perspective (Schipper 1984; Schou and Hewison 1999; NICE 2005).

Chaturvedi (1991) stated that the quality of *life* is not the same as the quality of *function*. What seems to be missing from quality of life assessment in cancer is a sense of *meaning* of the experience of cancer and treatment for an individual. The term 'meaning' gives some depth to functionality, but is not merely an extension of functionality. Meaning can include issues of understanding and acknowledgement from professionals and ideas about support (or non-support) from professionals or others, the nature of choice in treatment and the different experiences of the treatment trajectory or even treatment cessation. Such support is given by many members of the patient support network such as family, friends or professionals. There have been authors who supported a shift from the 'distress' model of psycho-oncology towards a positive exploration of the meaning in the experience of cancer and treatment (Fife 1995).

The psychological aspects of quality of life have been heavily linked to function and coping strategies. Using this method has resulted in assessing stress or distress felt by the patient with respect to diagnosis, treatment or prognosis and not assessing quality of life (Schou and Hewison 1999). Again the influence of the biomedical model arising from pathology is clear and so is its origin in the Cartesian philosophy of the body as a machine (Bowling 1997). Studies available in the literature (Speigel 1997; Schou and Hewison 1999) have examined various aspects of psychological response and 'functionality' in this way.

In the cancer literature outside of lung cancer (for example, breast and gynaecological cancers) there is a wealth of literature examining reaction to treatment, reaction to prognosis or diagnosis, self-esteem and sexuality but little literature on the health care context such as professional–patient relationships that have positively affected information giving in terms of optimism or pessimism (Speigel 1997). It can be said then that quality of life in the cancer literature is still based in terms of a functional approach that gives conventional biomedical perspectives priority. Such an approach would seem to fail to take account of the personal experience of people with cancer. Patients' experience of treatment, of the health care system and of living with cancer are all aspects of the social experience of illness.

The exploration of issues such as the effect of cancer on the individual and the group is now often termed psycho-oncology or psychosocial oncology, a discipline that has developed as a subspecialty of oncology over the last forty years as psychological factors have been seen to influence the experience of people with cancer (Holland 1998).

Lung cancer is an area where quality of life assessment has had an impact. As was seen earlier, many patients with lung cancer present in the advanced stages of the disease and there is limited benefit from most treatments in terms of quantity of life, so advanced lung cancer is seen as disease that is often treated in a palliative setting.

Quality of life in lung cancer

Despite the work of Karnofsky in the 1940s (Karnofsky 1948) until recently very little was written about the quality of life of people with lung cancer of any type. From the mid 1990s papers began to appear that reviewed and supported the idea that quality of life should be an end point in such studies (Kosmidis 1996; Hopwood and Thatcher 1990; Gralla 1994). These studies often employed a medical and pathological perspective. It has been noted by scholars (Stegbaur 1994; Cooley 1998) that there is a notable lack of theoretical quality-of-life work in the lung cancer patient population. The recent work on quality of life is driven by the cancer modernisation agenda, but it still centres on clinical trials and health-related quality of life measures that are essentially functional (NICE 2005).

Since the late 1980s the evolution of the definition of quality of life in lung cancer, particularly in non-small-cell lung cancer (NSCLC) became much more apparent. Upon reviewing the literature, a definite shift can be found to a more global approach and a broadening of health-related quality of life. From the mid 1980s the focus of investigation shifted from functioning and physical symptoms to a more global approach.

There has been an emerging consensus that there are at least four major dimensions of quality of life in advanced lung cancer that relate to health, including functional status, physical symptoms, emotional function and social function.

- **Functional status** is defined by normal day-to-day living activities and then further subdivisions of this with respect to performing the everyday activities of daily living such as bathing and dressing and role responsibilities such shopping and working. *Antecedents for functional status:* chemotherapy, co-morbidity, income, kilocalorie status, prior weight loss, time since surgery (Bakker *et al.* 1986; Sarna *et al.* 1993).
- **Physical symptoms** are the physical symptoms of the disease or treatment that is referred to. *Antecedents for physical symptoms:* chemotherapy, co-morbidity, gender, income, no surgical treatment, age, stage of disease, smoking, kilocalorie status, prior weight loss (Bakker *et al.* 1986; Sarna 1993).
- **Emotional function** refers to the affect, which includes positive and negative, for example depression and anxiety (Cella 1989). *Antecedents for emotional function:* age, spousal support, family support, time since diagnosis (Sarna 1993; Quinn *et al.* 1986).
- **Social function**: Schipper *et al.* (1990) referred to the maintenance of relationships with family and friends. Some authors maintain that this dimension has been under-used (Schipper *et al.* 1990). *Antecedents for social function:* age, marital status, family support (Sarna 1993).

As a result of this work, a definition of quality of life in advanced NSCLC was proposed by Mary Cooley:

> Quality of life in the context of NSCLC is the impact of the disease and/or treatment on the functional status, physical symptoms, affective state and interpersonal relationships as evaluated by the person with cancer.
>
> (Cooley 1998)

Cooley argued that an obvious antecedent for self-perceived quality of life is that an individual must have the ability 'to make a cognitive appraisal of his or her life'. In a study on quality of life and self-care in lung cancer (John 2010), patients cited family and social support, functional independence, physical well-being and spirituality as important aspects of quality of life. They identified fatigue as the factor most negatively affecting quality of life. Self-care strategies identified to improve quality of life were primarily related to fatigue management. Rest was the primary self-care strategy reportedly recommended by health care providers, but this strategy was ineffective. Helpful self-care strategies included budgeting time and energy, maintaining contact with family and friends for support and prayer (John 2010). This demonstrates the need for holistic assessment and good symptom control along with psychosocial support in patients with lung cancer.

Quality of life in advanced lung cancer: instruments used to measure health-related quality of life

Since the 1970s it has been common to use performance status as a prognostic indicator in lung cancer practice (Montezari et al. 1998). This arose from Carlens' Vitagram (Carlens et al. 1970) used to plot survival against performance status. Studies over the next twenty years appeared to confirm this proxy relationship (Montezari et al. 1998) demonstrating that performance status is a good predictor of quality of life, or rather an indicator of psychological, physical or symptom distress (Montezari et al. 1998). Although using performance status as a proxy for quality of life has been controversial, studies have shown correlation between performance status and global quality of life in some populations of lung cancer patients (Osoba et al. 1994). In practice, performance status continues to be used as a proxy for more thorough quality of life assessment (Montezari et al. 1998; Tishelman et al. 2000) and some authors caution against its continued use as a proxy, having made direct comparisons in patient groups (Koller et al. 2000).

Instruments used in lung cancer include:

- *Lung Cancer Symptom Scale (LCSS).* This instrument was developed in the 1980s at the Memorial Sloan-Kettering Cancer Center in the USA. It was based on an empirical conceptual model insofar as the LCSS attempts to depict to the quality-of-life dimensions or domains associated with the symptoms and, subsequently, the treatment and palliation of lung cancer (Hollen et al. 1994). Essentially, the LCSS examined the physical and functional aspects of quality of life, focusing on the major lung cancer symptoms and the effect of the symptoms on function and performance status.
- *The Functional Assessment of Cancer Therapy (FACT) lung version* is a self-reported 44-item questionnaire that is divided into two parts. The first part is a 34-item general/oncology-based health-related quality of life survey and the second part, consisting of 10 items, is lung cancer specific. The focus of the items in part two is a measure of lung cancer-related symptoms.
- *European Organisation for the Treatment of Cancer (EORTC) Quality of life questionnaire (QLQ).* The EORTC QLQ instrument evolved as a result of a desire by the EORTC to evaluate interventions in cancer therapies. A study group on quality of life was initiated by the EORTC in 1980 to develop a brief and practical quality of life measure (Aaronson 1991). The group developed the original 42-item questionnaire that used self-report. This was reduced to 36 items in the early 1990s (Aaronson 1991).The version in common use is a multidimensional questionnaire encompassing five functional domains (physical, role, cognitive, emotional and social) three symptom domains (nausea and vomiting, pain and fatigue) and single items such as a self-rating

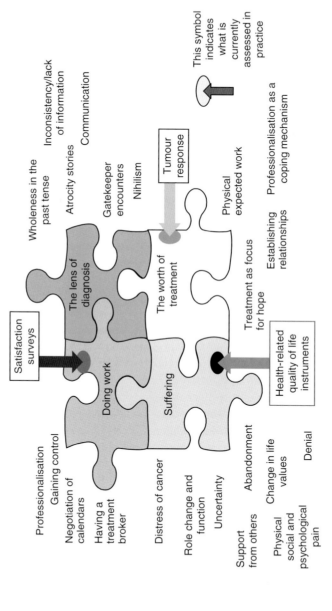

Fig. 9.2 The comparative properties of quality of life in patients receiving chemotherapy for advanced NSCLC.

visual analogue scale (VAS) of own quality of life. Patients rate each item using the terms 'not at all', 'a little', 'quite a bit' and 'very much'. It also includes a self-rated global VAS (Aaronson *et al.* 1993). In recent years a lung cancer site-specific module has been added that examines physical symptoms of lung cancer from a biomedical perspective.

Although there are limitations to these methods, quality of life scoring reveals interesting insights. A recent study in the USA examined the added value of quality of life as a prognostic factor for overall survival in patients with locally advanced non-small-cell lung cancer treated with chemoradiation therapy. The results of this study demonstrated that the baseline quality of life score replaced other indicators as the sole predictor of long-term over-all survival for patients with locally advanced NSCLC (Movsas *et al.* 2009). Even though quality of life scoring may give only a partial picture of quality of life globally, its measurement using validated tools seems to be worthwhile. A fuller comparison of what is currently assessed against global quality of life in patients receiving chemotherapy for NSCLC is shown in Figure 9.2.

Summary

Quality of life as an academic concept is still young. Although the classical theorists and philosophers have discussed the idea of quality of life and the good life for centuries, as an academic area of study in the reductionist sense it is surrounded by 'conceptual confusion' (Rapley 2003). This confusion can also been seen in attempts to clarify the conceptual confusion about quality of life. However, health-related quality of life can be a useful indicator in cancer care.

References

Aaronson, N.K., Ahmedazi, S. and Bullinger, M. (1991) The EORTC quality of care questionnaire. Interim results of an international field study. In: *Effect of Cancer on Quality of Life* (ed. D. Osoba).CRC Press, Boca Raton.

Aaronson, N.K., Ahmedazi, S., Bergman, B., *et al.* (1993) The EORTC QLQ-30 A qual-ity of life instrument for use in international trials in clinical oncology, *Journal of the National Cancer Institute*, **85**, 365–376.

Bakker, W., van Ooserom A.T., Aaronson, N.K., van Breukelen, F.J., Bins, M.C., Hermans, J. (1986) Vindistine, cisplatin and bleomycin combination chemo-therapy in non small-cell lung cancer: survival and quality of life. *European Journal of Cancer and Clinical Oncology*, **22**, 963–970.

Berckman, K.L. and Austin, J.K. (1993) The causal attribution and perceived control and adjustment in patients with lung cancer. *Oncology Nursing Forum*, **20**, 20–30.

Bowling, A. (1997) *Measuring Health*, 2nd edn. Open University Press, Buckingham.

Bowling, A. (2003) Current state of the art in quality of life measurement. In: *Quality Of Life* (eds Carr, A., Higginson, I. and Robinson, P.G), pp. 1–18. BMJ, London.

Bullinger, M., Anderson, R., Cella, D.F. and Aaronson, N.K. (1993) Developing and evaluating cross-cultural instruments-from minimum requirements to optimum models. *Quality of Life Research*, **2**, 451-459.

Cancer Services Collaborative (2001) *Service Improvement Guide (lung)*. HMSO, London.

Carlens, E., Dahlström, G. and Nöu, E. (1970) Comparative survival of lung cancer patients after diagnosis. *Scandinavian Journal of Respiratory Disease*, **51**, 268-275.

Carr, A., Gibson, B. and Robinson, P.G. (2001) Is quality of life determined by expectation or experience? *British Medical Journal*, **322**, 1240-1243.

Cassell, E.J. (2004) *The Nature of Suffering and the Goals of Medicine*, 2nd edn. Oxford University Press, Oxford.

Cella, D.F. (1989) Functional assessment and quality of life: Current views on measurement and intervention. American Cancer Society. *First National Conference on Cancer Nursing Research*, 1989, Atlanta.

Chapple, A., Ziebland, S. and McPherson, A. (2004) Stigma, shame and blame experienced by patients with lung cancer: qualitative study. *British Medical Journal*, **328** (7454): 1470. doi:10.1136/bmj.38111.639734.7c. 2004.

Chaturvedi, S.K. (1991) What's important for quality of life to Indians – in relation to cancer. *Social Science and Medicine*, **33** (1), 91-94.

Cicero (Grant, M. transl.) (1971) *On the Good Life*. Penguin, Harmondsworth.

Cooley, M.E. (1998) Quality of life in persons with non small-cell lung cancer-a concept analysis, *Cancer Nursing*, **21** (3), 151-161.

Corner, J. (1997) Beyond survival rates and side effects: cancer nursing as therapy. The Robert Tiffany Lecture. *Cancer Nursing*, **20** (1), 3-11.

de Haes, J.C and Van Knippenberg, F.C.E. (1985) Quality of life of cancer patients: a review of the literature. *Social Science and Medicine*, **20** (8), 809-817.

DH (2000a) *The NHS Cancer Plan: A Plan for Investment, A Plan for Reform*. HMSO, London.

DH (2000b) *The Nursing Contribution to Cancer Care*, HMSO, London.

DH (2003) *The NHS Cancer Plan – Maintaining the momentum*, HMSO.

DH (2007) *Cancer Reform Strategy*. HMSO, London.

Faull, C. and Woof, R. (2002) *Palliative Care*. Oxford University Press, Oxford.

Fife, B.L. (1995) The measurement of meaning in illness. *Social Science and Medicine*, **40** (8), 1021-1028.

Gralla, R.J. (1994) Measuring quality of life in patients with lung cancer. *Lung Cancer*, **11**, 70-71.

Houldin, A.D. (2000) *Patients with Cancer*. Lippincott, Philadelphia.

Holland, J.C. (1998) *Psycho-oncology*. Lippincott, Philadelphia.

Hollen, P.J., Gralla, R.J., Kris, M.G., *et al*. (1994) Measurement of quality of life in patients with lung cancer in multicenter trials of new therapies. *Cancer*, **73** (8), 2087-2098.

Hopwood, P. and Thatcher, N. (1990) Preliminary experience with quality of life evaluation in patients with lung cancer. *Oncology*, **4**, 158-162.

John, L.D. (2010) Self-care strategies used by patients with lung cancer to promote quality of life. *Oncology Nursing Forum*, **37** (3), 339-347.

Karnofsky, D.A., Abelman, W.H., Craver, L.F. and Burchenal, J.H. (1948) The use of nitrogen mustard in the palliative treatment of carcinoma, with particular reference to bronchogenic carcinoma. *Cancer*, **1**, 634-656.

Kosmidis, P. (1996) Quality of life as a new endpoint. *Chest*, **109**, 110s-112s.

Koller, M., Lorentz, W., Wagner, K., *et al*. (2000) Expectations and quality of life of cancer patients undergoing radiotherapy. *Journal of the Royal Society of Medicine*, **93** (12), 609-610.

Koller, M. and Lorentz, W. (2002) Quality of life a deconstruction for clinicians, *Journal of the Royal Society of Medicine*, **95**, 481-488.

Krishnasamy, M. and Wilkie, E. (1999) *Lung Cancer: Pateints', Families' and Professionals' Perceptions of Health Care Need. A National Needs Assessment Study*. Macmillan Practice Development Unit, London.

Leary, A. and Corrigan, P. (2005) Redesign of thoracic surgical services-using an on oncology focus to inform change. *European Journal of Oncology Nursing*, **9** (1), 74-78.

Maslow, A. (1954) *Motivation and Personality*. Harper, New York.

Mast, M.E. (1998) Adult uncertainty and illness: a critical review of the literature. *Scholarly Inquiry for Nursing Practice*, **9** (1), 3-29.

Mathiesen, C.M. and Stam, H.J. (1995) Re-negotiating identity: cancer narratives. *Sociology of Health and Illness*, **15** (3), 283-306.

Meeberg, G.A. (1993) Quality of life: a concept analysis. *Journal of Advanced Nursing*, **18**, 32-38.

Montezari, A., Gillis, C. and McEwen, J. (1998) Quality of life in patients with lung cancer: a review of the literature from 1970-1995. *Chest*, **113** (2), 467-481.

Movsas, B., Moughan, J., Sarna, L., *et al.* (2009) Quality of life supersedes the classic prognosticators for long-term survival in locally advanced non-small-cell lung cancer: an analysis of RTOG 9801. *Journal of Clinical Oncology*, **27** (34), 5816-5822.

NICE (2005) *The Diagnosis and Treatment of Lung Cancer*. National Institute for Clinical Excellence and National Collaborating Centre for Acute Care, London.

Oxford English Dictionary (1995) Oxford University Press, Oxford.

Osoba, D., Murray, N. and Gelmon, K. (1994) Quality of life and weight change in patients receiving dose-intensive chemotherapy. *Oncology*, **8**, 61-65.

Parsons, T. (1951) *The Social System*. Free Press, New York.

Quinn, M.E., Fontana, A.F. and Reznikoff, M. (1986) Psychological distress in reaction to lung cancer as a function of spousal support and coping strategy. *Journal of Psychosocial Oncology*, **4**, 79-90.

Rapley, M. (2003) *Quality Of Life Research*. Sage, London.

Sarna, L. (1993) Correlates of symptom distress in women with lung cancer. *Cancer Practice*, **1**, 21-28.

Sarna, L., Lindsey, A.M., Dean, H., Brecht, M.L. and McCorkle, R. (1993) Nutritional intake, weight change, symptom distress and functional status over time in adults with lung cancer. *Oncology Nursing Forum*, **20**, 481-489.

Scambler, G. (1991) *Sociology As Applied To Medicine*, 3rd edn. Ballière Tindall, London.

Schipper, H., Clinch, J., McMurray, A. and Levitt, M. (1984) Measuring quality of life in cancer patients – the Functional Living Index-Cancer: development and validation. *Journal of Clinical Oncology*, **2** (5), 472-483.

Schipper, H., Clinch, J., Powell, V. (1990) Definition and quality of life conceptual issues. In: *Quality of Life Assessments in Clinical Trials* (ed. B. Spiker). Raven Press, New York.

Schou, K.C. and Hewison, J. (1999) *Experiencing Cancer*. Open University Press, Buckingham.

Speigel, D. (1997) Psychosocial aspects of breast cancer treatment. *Seminars in Oncology*, **24**(1 Suppl. 1), s1.36-s1.47.

Stegbaur, C.C. (1994) *Expanding a grounded theory: the latent theory of quality of life in older men with non small-cell lung cancer*, PhD thesis, University of Texas.

Stetz, K.M., Haberman, H.R., Holcombe, J. and Jones, S. (1995) Oncology Nursing Society research priority survey. *Oncology Nursing Forum*, **22**, 785-790.

Tishelman, C., Degner, L.F. and Mueller, B. (2000) Measuring symptom distress in patients with lung cancer. *Cancer Nursing*, **2**, 82-90.

WHO (1993) *WHOQoL Study Protocol*. World Health Organization, Geneva (MNH7PSF/93.9).

Wulff, H. (1999) The two cultures of medicine: objective facts versus subjectivity and values. [Editorial]. *Journal of the Royal Society of Medicine*, **92**, 549-552.

Index

ACTH *see* adrenocorticotrophic hormone
active listening 149-50, 151
activities of daily living (ADL) 190, 196
activity planning 132
acute pain 169
adenocarcinoma 6-7
  chemotherapy 54-5
  presentation and diagnosis 16, 21, 26,
    29-30
  supportive care 153
ADH *see* antidiuretic hormone
adjuvant treatment
  chemotherapy 51-2
  end-of-life care 171-5
  surgical interventions 108-10
ADL *see* activities of daily living
adrenocorticotrophic hormone
    (ACTH) 24
adult cardiac surgery 88
advanced NSCLC 50, 53-5, 197-9
age-related incidence rates 3
agitation 178-9
alkaline phosphatase (ALP) 20
anaesthesia
  quality of life 190
  surgical interventions 91, 107, 113
analgesia
  end-of-life care 163-4, 171-4
  nursing care 127-9, 134
  quality of life 190-1
  surgical interventions 107, 113
analgesic ladder 128, 172-3
anorexia 25, 130, 154-5
antiangiogenics 55-6
anticoagulants 133
anticonvulsants 175
antidepressants 175
antidiuretic hormone (ADH) 24
antiemetics 172, 174
anti-epidermal growth factor
    receptors 56
antiepileptics 129
antimuscarinics 178-9

antispasmodics 175
anxiety
  nursing care 129-30, 136
  supportive care 147, 150
anxiolytics 129-30
appetite disruption 130-1, 154-5
arsenic 27
asbestos exposure
  mesothelioma 43-4
  presentation and diagnosis 26
asthma 18
attitudes towards cancer 148-9, 151
autofluorescence bronchoscopy 34

benefit of the doubt concept 92
benefits rights 153
benzodiazepines 129-30, 176
beryllium 27
bevacizumab 55
bilateral thoracotomy 107
bilirubin 20
bilobectomy 105-6
biological agents 49, 52, 57, 60-1
biopsies
  presentation and diagnosis 28-30,
    35-8, 45
  surgical interventions 90, 100-3
bisphosphonates 129, 134
blood tests 45-6
bone metastases
  presentation and diagnosis 21, 24, 31-2
  radiotherapy 79-80
bone pain 171
BPF *see* bronchopleural fistulae
brachytherapy 68, 79
brain metastases 79
breakthrough pain 169
breast cancer 154
breathlessness
  end-of-life care 174-7
  nursing care 129-30
  presentation and diagnosis 18, 19
  surgical interventions 111, 114-15

Lung Cancer: A Multidisciplinary Approach, First Edition. Edited by Alison Leary.
© 2012 Blackwell Publishing Ltd. Published 2012 by Blackwell Publishing Ltd.

bronchoalveolar cell cancer 112
bronchopleural fistulae (BPF) 113
bronchoscopy
    presentation and diagnosis 29-31, 34-5
    surgical interventions 90, 101
bulky Hodgkin disease 65-6

cachexia 25, 130, 154-5
calcitonin 24
cancer cachexia syndrome (CCS) 25, 130,
    154-5
Cancer Reform Strategy 8, 122-4
cancer services 8-11
carboplatin 50-1, 54-9
carcinoid tumours 7, 111-12
carcinoma in situ 34
cardiopulmonary complications 95-6
cardiothoracic surgery 88
cardiovascular risks 98
caregivers 152-3, 155
CCS see cancer cachexia syndrome
central tumours 19-20
cerebellar degeneration 24-5
cetuximab 56-7
CHART see continuous hyperfractionated
    accelerated radiotherapy
chemotherapy 49-64
    adjuvant treatment 51-2
    advanced NSCLC 50, 53-5
    end-of-life care 171
    mesothelioma 59-61
    neo-adjuvant treatment 52-3
    non-small-cell lung cancer 49-50, 51-7
    patient-related factors 50
    quality of life 191, 198
    radiotherapy 75, 76-8
    side effects and toxicity 50, 51
    small-cell lung cancer 49-50, 57-9
    supportive care 148, 153
    surgical interventions 106-7, 108-10
    targeted therapies 55-7
chest drains 114
chest pain 17
chest radiography (CXR)
    presentation and diagnosis 16, 19, 27,
        28-9, 44-5
    surgical interventions 93-4
choline-PET 33-4
chromium 27
chronic obstructive pulmonary disease
    (COPD) 18-20, 26
chronic pain 169
chylothorax 115
cisplatin 50-61
clinical nurse specialists (CNS) 11, 155
clinical target volume (CTV) 71-2
CNS see clinical nurse specialists

coagulopathy paraneoplastic
    syndromes 23
communicating the diagnosis/prognosis
    147-8, 156
computed tomography (CT)
    presentation and diagnosis 16, 20, 21,
        28-31, 33, 41-2, 44-5
    radiotherapy 66-7, 70-1
    surgical interventions 93-4, 105-6
connective tissue paraneoplastic
    syndromes 23
constitutional paraneoplastic
    syndromes 25-6
continuous hyperfractionated
    accelerated radiotherapy
    (CHART) 74, 75-6
continuous subcutaneous infusion
    (CSCI) 177-80
COPD see chronic obstructive pulmonary
    disease
coping strategies 151, 153, 194-5
coronary artery bypass surgery 98
corticosteroids 130, 175
cough 17, 131-2
counselling 136, 152
critical nursing behaviours 180-1
CSCI see continuous subcutaneous
    infusion
CT see computed tomography
CTV see clinical target volume
cultural factors
    end-of-life care 180
    supportive care 148-9, 154
cutaneous paraneoplastic syndromes 23
CXR see chest radiography
cyclophosphamide 53
cytopathology 45

death rattle 179
dehydration at end-of-life 164
delivery of cancer services 8-11
depression
    nursing care 136
    supportive care 147, 150
diagnosis see presentation
    and diagnosis
diamorphine 177, 179
diaphragm reconstruction 105-6
dietary factors
    nursing care 130-1, 132
    supportive care 154-5
disease-specific information 11-13
diuretics 133
docetaxel 50-1
dose volume histograms (DVH) 73
dysphagia 18, 20, 177
dyspnoea 19, 95, 99

Eastern Co-operative Oncology Group
(ECOG) score 27
EBUS see endobronchial ultrasound
ECOG see Eastern Co-operative Oncology
Group
EGFR see epidermal growth factor
receptors
emotional factors
patient needs assessment 125-7, 135-6,
147-8, 150-2
quality of life 191, 196
emphysema 96, 98
empyema 113
end-of-life care
breathlessness 174-7
context 159
definitions 160
dehydration versus rehydration 164
diagnosing dying 162-3
dying in the twenty-first century 160-2
ethics 163-4, 165
health professionals' attitudes to the
dying 161-2
historical context 159-60
last hours 177-81
nursing care 124
pain management 163-4, 168-74
planning care for the dying
patient 164-81
social care 180-1
supportive care 154, 156
symptom management 163, 166-8
see also palliative care
endobronchial ultrasound (EBUS)
35-6, 42
endocrine paraneoplastic syndromes
23, 24
endoscopic ultrasound (EUS) 35-6, 42
environmental carcinogens 5-6, 27
EORTC see European Organisation for
the Treatment of Cancer
epidemiology 1-6
ethnicity 5
social deprivation 2-4
supportive care 153-4
tobacco smoking 1, 4-5, 15-16, 191
epidermal growth factor receptors
(EGFR) 56
epidural analgesia 107
epirubicin 58
erlotinib 56
ethics 163-4, 165
ethnicity 5
etiology of lung cancer 2-6
environmental and industrial
carcinogens 5-6
radon gas 5

social deprivation 2-4
tobacco smoking 1, 4-5
etoposide 51-3, 57-9
European Organisation for the Treatment
of Cancer (EORTC) 197-8
EUS see endoscopic ultrasound
euthanasia 163, 164
exercise 129, 132
extensive stage SCLC 58-9
external beam radiotherapy 68
extrapleural analgesia 107
extrapulmonary intrathoracic
disease 18-20
extrathoracic disease 20-2

FACT see Functional Assessment of
Cancer Therapy
family members
end-of-life care 161, 165, 180-1
nursing care 121-2, 135-7
quality of life 194
supportive care 148, 152-3, 155
fatigue 50, 131, 132
FDG see [18F]fluorodeoxyglucose
fear of death 161-2
FEV_1 see forced expiratory volume in 1
second
fine-needle aspiration (FNA) 31, 35
fitness for surgery 92-3, 97-8
five-year survival 2, 194
[18F]fluorodeoxyglucose (FDG) PET 32-4
FNA see fine-needle aspiration
forced expiratory volume in 1 second
(FEV_1)
presentation and diagnosis 18, 35, 41-2
radiotherapy 74
surgical interventions 95-8, 105
frozen section 100-1
Functional Assessment of Cancer
Therapy (FACT) 197
functional quality of life 194-5, 196

gamma-glutamyl transferase 20
gefitinib 56
gemcitabine 50-1, 54-5, 58-9
gender factors 2-3
gross tumour volume (GTV) 71-2

haemological paraneoplastic
syndromes 23
haemoptysis 17
histopathology 45
hope 148, 151
Horner syndrome 19
hospice movement 159-60, 182
HPOA see hypertrophic pulmonary
osteoarthropathy

humanising the hospital setting 182
hypercalcaemia 24
hypertrophic pulmonary
    osteoarthropathy (HPOA) 22-3
hyponatraemia 24
hypoxia 129-30

ifosfamide 52, 54, 58
IGF-1R *see* insulin-like growth factor
    receptor type 1
impaired lung function 93-7
IMRT *see* intensity modulated
    radiotherapy
inappropriate secretion of antidiuretic
    hormone (ISADH) 7
incidental N2 disease (IIIA2) 108-9
industrial carcinogens 5-6, 26-7, 43-4
information needs 11-13
insulin-like growth factor receptor type 1
    (IGF-1R) 57
intensity modulated radiotherapy
    (IMRT) 67
intercostal analgesia 107
interstitial lung disease 95
intracranial tumours 21
intra-parenchymal lesions 16
intrapulmonary disease 17-18
intravenous fluids 164
invasive biopsies 100
irinotecan 59
ISADH *see* inappropriate secretion of
    antidiuretic hormone

Karnofsky scores 27, 50, 60

Lambert-Eaton myasthenic syndrome
    (LEMS) 24-5
large-cell carcinoma 7
last hours care 177-81
laxatives 172, 174
LCP *see* Liverpool Care Pathway
LCSS *see* Lung Cancer Symptom Scale
left pneumonectomy 93-7
LEMS *see* Lambert-Eaton myasthenic
    syndrome
levomepromazine 176
lifestyle modifications 153
limited stage SCLC 58
linear accelerators 66, 68-9
Liverpool Care Pathway (LCP) 166-7
low mood 135-6
Lung Cancer Symptom Scale (LCSS) 197
lung fibrosis 83
lung radiotherapy *see* radiotherapy
lung transplantation 90
lung volume reduction surgery (LVRS)
    effect 98

lymph nodes
    nursing care 133
    presentation and diagnosis 19, 20,
        30-3, 35-41
    radiotherapy 74
    surgical interventions 104
lymphadenectomy 108

Macmillan Cancer Information
    Centres 12-13
magnetic resonance imaging (MRI)
    21, 31, 45
malignant pleural mesothelioma 7-8, 59
malnutrition 154-5
MDT *see* multidisciplinary teams
mediastinal lymph node maps 37
mediastinal lymphadenopathy 28, 30-1
mediastinal radiotherapy 58
mediastinoscopy 35, 90, 101
mediastinotomy 90, 102
medical linear accelerators 68-9
mesothelioma 7-8
    asbestos exposure 43-4
    chemotherapy 59-61
    clinical features 43
    investigations 44-6
    presentation and diagnosis 42-6
    referral to specialists 44
    staging 46
metastases
    chemotherapy 52, 59
    non-small-cell lung cancer 6
    nursing care 127-9, 134
    presentation and diagnosis 19, 20-2,
        24, 28-33, 38-41
    radiotherapy 79-80
    small-cell lung cancer 7
    surgical interventions 109-10
MI *see* myocardial infarction
microinvasive carcinomas 34
mini-thoracotomy 90, 103
mitomycin 52, 54, 60-1
monoclonal antibodies 57
morphine 129-30, 172-3, 176-7
MRI *see* magnetic resonance imaging
multidisciplinary teams (MDT) 8-11
    clinical nurse specialist role 11
    complexity of cancer care 9-11
    coordinator role 11
    end-of-life care 162-3
    nursing care 121-2, 137
    quality of life 190
    radiotherapy 70
    supportive care 146, 147
    surgical interventions 88-92, 94-6,
        112, 115
multileaf collimators 67, 69

musculoskeletal paraneoplastic
   syndromes 22-3
myelosuppression 51, 59
myocardial infarction (MI) 98

N2 disease 108-9
natural history of untreated cancer
   16-17
navelbine 52
neo-adjuvant treatment 52-3, 106-7
nephrotoxicity 51
nerve injury 114
neuroendocrine cancer 111-12
neurological paraneoplastic
   syndromes 23, 24-5
neuropathic pain 128-9, 171
neuropathic side effects 51
neutropenic septicaemia 50
non-opioid analgesia 171-4
non-small-cell lung cancer (NSCLC) 6-7
   advanced 50, 53-5
   chemotherapy 49-50, 51-7
   epidemiology 2
   nursing care 133
   presentation and diagnosis 16, 32-3,
      38-40, 41-2
   quality of life 195-6, 197-9
   radiotherapy 73-6
   staging 38-40, 41-2
   surgical interventions 100, 108-10,
      111-12
non-verbal indicators of pain 170
NRS see numerical rating scales
NSCLC see non-small-cell lung cancer
numerical rating scales (NRS) 128, 170
nursing care 121-44
   breathlessness 129-30
   challenges of lung cancer 124-37
   cough 131-2
   end-of-life care 167, 180-1
   family members 121-2, 135-7
   fatigue 131, 132
   healthcare settings 121-2
   important issues 122
   low mood 135-6
   multidisciplinary teams 121-2, 137
   pain management 127-9, 134
   palliative care 138-9
   patient needs assessment 125-7, 135-7
   patient-reported problems 126-37
   poor appetite 130-1
   quality of life 193-4
   specialist nurses 138-9
   spinal cord compression 133-5
   superior vena cava obstruction 132-3
   UK context 123-4
nutritional supplementation 130-1, 155

oat cell see small-cell lung cancer
oesophageal stricture 83
oesophagitis 81
open surgery 107
operability 92-3, 97-8
opioids 129-30, 163-4, 171-4, 176-7
OS see overall survival
out-patients 146
overall survival (OS) 75-6
oxygen therapy 129-30, 175-6
oxytocin 24

paclitaxel 50-1, 54-6
paediatric cardiac surgery 88
pain management
   end-of-life care 163-4, 168-74
   nursing care 127-9, 134
   surgical interventions 107, 113
pain relief ladder 128, 172-3
palliative care 159-87
   breathlessness 174-7
   context 159
   definitions 160
   dehydration versus rehydration 164
   diagnosing dying 162-3
   dying in the twenty-first century 160-2
   ethics 163-4, 165
   health professionals' attitudes to the
      dying 161-2
   historical context 159-60
   last hours 177-81
   nursing care 124, 138-9
   pain management 163-4, 168-74
   planning care for the dying
      patient 164-81
   radiotherapy 70, 72-4, 78-80, 171
   social care 180-1
   supportive care 148, 154, 156
   surgical interventions 110-11
   symptom management 163, 166-8, 182
Pancoast tumours 19, 106-7
Papworth Thoracic Surgery Unit 99
paraneoplastic syndromes 22-6
parathyroid hormone-related peptide
   (PTH-rP) 24
paravertebral analgesia 107
parenchymal opacity 30
passive euthanasia 164
pathological diagnosis 100-1
patient-centred approach to care 145-6
patient-centred decision making 89
patient-controlled analgesia (PCA) 107,
   113
patient information 11-13
patient needs assessment 125-7, 135-7,
   147-8, 149-52
patient positioning 70-1

patients' attitudes towards cancer 148-9, 151
PCA *see* patient-controlled analgesia
PCI *see* prophylactic cranial irradiation
peak expiratory flow (PEF) 18
pemetrexed 51, 54-5, 60-1
performance status 27
pericardial effusions 111
perioperative death 95
peripheral neuropathy 24-5
PET *see* positron emission tomography
phrenic nerve 19
physical needs assessment 125-7
physical quality of life 196
planning target volume (PTV) 72-3
pleural disease 20
pleural effusions
   presentation and diagnosis 28, 38, 44-5
   surgical interventions 110-11
pleural mesothelioma 7-8, 59
pneumonectomy 95, 97, 99, 108-9, 113-14
poor appetite 130-1
PORT *see* postoperative radiotherapy
positron emission tomography (PET) 21, 32-4, 41-2
postoperative complications 112-15
postoperative radiotherapy (PORT) 76
post-pneumonectomy pulmonary oedema 113-14
presentation and diagnosis 15-47
   algorithm for NSCLC 42
   clinical features 17-22
   extrapulmonary intrathoracic disease 18-20
   extrathoracic disease 20-2
   intrapulmonary disease 17-18
   investigation of lung cancer 28-38
   mesothelioma 42-6
   natural history of untreated cancer 16-17
   paraneoplastic syndromes 22-6
   performance status 27
   pleural effusions 28, 38, 44-5
   radiological investigations 28-34
   risk factors for lung cancer 26-7
   staging of lung cancer 33, 38-42, 46
   tissue confirmation investigations 34-8
prophylactic cranial irradiation (PCI) 58, 76, 77-8
prostate cancer 154
psychiatric/psychological interventions 136, 151-2
psychological factors
   needs assessment 125-7, 135-6, 147-8, 150-2
   quality of life 194-5

PTH-rP *see* parathyroid hormone-related peptide
PTV *see* planning target volume
pulmonary collapse 28
pulmonary function tests 46
pulmonary oedema 113-14, 164
pyramid model of pain relief 128-9

qualitative aspects of care 123
quality of life (QOL) 189-202
   advanced lung cancer 197-9
   chemotherapy 50, 54, 60
   definitions 189
   end-of-life care 159-60, 166, 168, 180
   functionality 194-5, 196
   measurement and assessment 192-4, 197-9
   nursing care 127, 135
   perceptions 190-2
   presentation and diagnosis 20, 25, 27
   psychological factors 194-5
   self-care strategies 196-7
   social ties 191-2
   supportive care 145, 150, 154, 156
   surgical interventions 90-1, 96, 110
   treatment calendar management 192
   treatment success 194
Quality of life questionnaire (QLQ) 197-8
quantitative aspects of care 123

R classification *see* resectability
radiation pneumonitis 74, 82-3
radical radiotherapy 70, 73-5, 80
radiofrequency ablation (RFA) 98
radionuclide bone scanning 31-2
radiotherapy 58, 65-86
   acute side effects 81-2
   beam arrangement 72-3
   brachytherapy 68, 79
   brain metastases 79
   cell kill mechanisms 67-8
   chemotherapy 75, 76-8
   continuous hyperfractionated accelerated radiotherapy 74, 75-6
   delivery methods 68
   end-of-life care 171
   historical context 65-7
   implementation and validation 73
   linear accelerators 66, 68-9
   long-term toxicity 82-3
   management of patients 80-3
   new techniques under evaluation 83-4
   non-small-cell lung cancer 73-6
   palliative 70, 72-4, 78-80
   patient positioning 70-1
   planning 69-70, 72-3

postoperative 76
preparation 70
principles 65-73
radiation pneumonitis 74, 82-3
radical 70, 73-5, 80
side effects and toxicity 80-1
small-cell lung cancer 76-8, 82
spinal cord compression and bony
   metastases 79-80
supportive care 148, 153
tumour localisation 71
tumour volume definition 71-2
whole-brain 82
radon gas 5, 27
raltitrexed 60
recurrent disease 110
recurrent focal pneumonia 17
recurrent laryngeal nerve palsy 19
referral to specialists
   mesothelioma 44
   nursing care 134
   surgical interventions 89
rehabilitation follow-up 112-15
rehydration at end-of-life 164
relaxation 129, 132
religious needs 180
renal paraneoplastic syndromes 23
resectability (R classification) 91-2
respiratory depressants 176-7
respiratory gating 83
respiratory tract secretions 179
RFA see radiofrequency ablation
risk stratification 98-9

SCC see spinal cord compression;
   squamous cell carcinoma
SCLC see small-cell lung cancer
sedatives 178-9
self-care strategies 196-7
serum mesothelin-related protein
   (SMRP) 45-6
SIADH see syndrome of inappropriate
   antidiuretic hormone
skin erythema 81
sleep disorders 132
sleeve resections 91
small-cell lung cancer (SCLC) 6, 7
   chemotherapy 49-50, 57-9
   extensive stage 58-9
   limited stage 58
   presentation and diagnosis 16, 18-19,
     21, 40-1
   radiotherapy 76-8, 82
   second-line treatment 59
   staging 40-1, 58-9
   surgical interventions 100, 112
smoking see tobacco smoking

SMRP see serum mesothelin-related
   protein
social attitudes towards cancer 148-9, 151
social care 180-1
social factors
   epidemiology 2-4
   needs assessment 125-7, 135-7
   quality of life 196
   supportive care 153-4
social ties 191-2
solitary pulmonary nodules 28-30
somatic pain 171
sorafenib 55-6
specialist nurses 11, 138-9, 155
spinal cord compression (SCC)
   nursing care 133-5
   presentation and diagnosis 21
   radiotherapy 79-80
spiritual needs 180
spirometry 97
sputum cytology 34
squamous cell carcinoma (SCC) 6
   presentation and diagnosis 16, 24, 26,
     29
   radiotherapy 75
   surgical interventions 105-6
staging of lung cancer
   chemotherapy 58-9
   nursing care 126-7
   presentation and diagnosis 33, 38-42,
     46
   surgical interventions 100, 102
step process to analgesia 128
stereotactic lung radiotherapy 83-4
steroids 133
stress management 153
stridor 18
suffering 191
superior vena caval obstruction (SVCO)
   nursing care 132-3
   presentation and diagnosis 18-19, 22, 27
supportive care 145-58
   attitudes towards cancer 148-9, 151
   communicating the diagnosis/
     prognosis 147-8, 156
   context 145-6
   family members 148, 152-3, 155
   improving the patient
     experience 153-6
   multidisciplinary teams 146, 147
   patient-centred approach 145-6
   psychological distress 147-8, 150-2
   uncertainty 149-50
surgical interventions 87-119
   adjuvant chemotherapy 106-7, 108-10
   anaesthesia 91, 107, 113
   benefit of the doubt concept 92

surgical interventions (*cont'd*)
  bronchoalveolar cell cancer 112
  carcinoid tumours and neuroendocrine
    cancer 111-12
  cardiovascular risks 98
  decision-making process 90-9
  forced expiratory volume in 1
    second 95-8, 105
  historical context 87-8
  left pneumonectomy case study 93-7
  lung resections with curative
    intent 101-3
  management of metastases 109-10
  multidisciplinary teams 88-92, 94-6,
    112, 115
  non-small-cell lung cancer 100, 108-10,
    111-12
  open surgery 107
  operability 92-3, 97-8
  outcomes 109
  pain management 107, 113
  palliative 110-11
  Papworth Thoracic Surgery Unit 99
  pathological diagnosis 100-1
  patient-centred decision making 89
  postoperative complications and
    follow-up 112-15
  postsurgical care 115
  recovery, discharge and
    mobilisation 107
  recurrent disease 110
  resectability 91-2
  risk stratification 98-9
  role of the surgeon 89-90
  small-cell lung cancer 100, 112
  staging of lung cancer 100, 102
  T descriptor 101-2, 105-7
  technical factors 90-1
  UK surgical resection rates 88-9
  video assisted thoracic surgery 90,
    103-5
surgical resection 2, 88-9, 91-2, 95-6,
  98, 101-7
SVCO *see* superior vena caval
  obstruction
symptom clusters 126
symptom management at end-of-life 163,
  166-8, 182
syndrome of inappropriate antidiuretic
  hormone (SIADH) 24
syringe drivers 177-80

T descriptor 101-2, 105-7
targeted therapies 55-7

TB *see* tuberculosis
TCA *see* tricyclic antidepressants
thalidomide 55, 58
thoracic irradiation (TI) 76, 77
thoracic surgery 87-8, 98-9
thoracotomy 36-8, 45
three-dimensional computed tomography
  (3D-CT) 66-7, 70-1
thrombolysis 133
TI *see* thoracic irradiation
tissue confirmation investigations 34-8
TNM staging 38-41, 102
tobacco smoking
  epidemiology 1, 4-5, 15-16
  quality of life 191
  risk factors 26
tracheal obstruction 18
transthoracic needle aspiration 35
treatment calendar management 192
tricyclic antidepressants (TCA) 129
tuberculosis (TB) 87
tumour localisation 71
tumour volume definition 71-2
tyrosine kinase inhibitors 56

ultrasonography 31, 35-6
uncertainty 149-50
unilateral thoracotomy 107

validated pain assessment tools 170
VAS *see* visual analogue scales
vascular endothelial growth factor
  (VEGF) 23
VATS *see* video-assisted thorascopic
  surgery
VEGF *see* vascular endothelial growth
  factor
verbal rating scales (VRS) 128, 170
video-assisted thorascopic surgery
  (VATS) 36-8, 45, 90, 103-5
vinblastine 51-2, 60-1
vincristine 51
vindesine 51-2
vinorelbine 50-2, 56-8, 61
visceral pain 171
visual analogue scales (VAS) 128,
  170, 199
vocal cord palsy 19
vocal indicators of pain 170
VRS *see* verbal rating scales

welfare rights 153
WHO pain relief ladder 128, 172-3
whole-brain radiotherapy 82